The Mechanism of Life

Illness as Part of Life's Journey

Katsumi Ishihara

いのちの仕組み
病むことも生きること。

石原克己

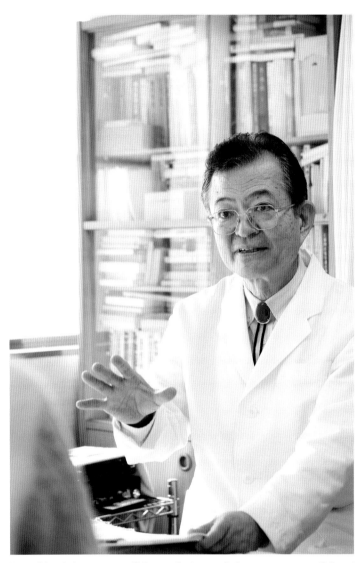

In traditional Japanese medicine, patient consultations are an essential part of treatment protocol to discover the root cause of an illness. Careful attention is given to the patient's general concerns regarding work, lifestyle, or family relationships.

伝統医療において面談は病の原因を探るための重要な時間。治療者は相談者の症状だけではなく、生活の仕方や悩み、家族関係などにも関心を向け、真剣に耳を傾ける

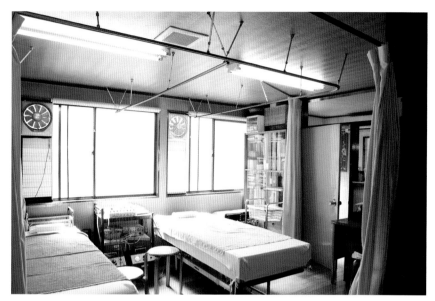

Dr. Kazumi Ishihara's clinic in Goi, in Chiba Prefecture. Adjacent to the hari-kyu ('acupuncture and moxibustion') clinic is a kampo ('Sino-Japanese') traditional medicine pharmacy.

千葉県市原市五井にある著者の診療所。鍼灸の治療所の隣に漢方薬局が併設されている

Various kinds of needles used for treat-ment are stored in a sterilizer machine. Dr. Ishihara selects the needles to be used in response to the patient's symptoms and phase of treatment.

治療に使う様々な鍼が滅菌器に保管されている。著者は患者の症状、治療の段階に合わせてその都度適切な鍼を選び直して使う

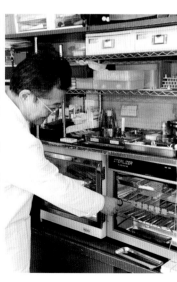

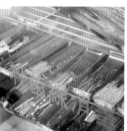

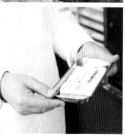

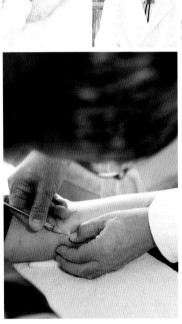

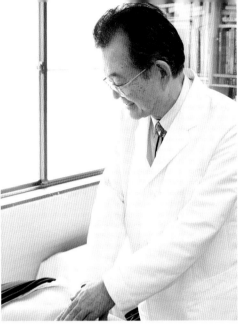

↑Examining the condition of the organs by palpation.

触診で内臓の状態を感知する

←Healing a sprain injury in the left elbow.Reliving stagnation in the affected area by using a special needle called zashi-shin ('pricking needle') to stimulate subcutaneous tissue.

ヒジの捻挫の治療にあたる。挫刺鍼(ざししん)という鍼を使い、皮下の線維に刺激を与えることで患部の鬱滞をとっていく

Needles are not the only healing modality used for hari-kyu treatment. Cupping therapy is used to stimulate subcutaneous tissue by local suction on the skin (left). Another widely used method is moxibustion, a form of thermotherapy in which moxa ('dried mugwort') is burned on acupuncture points along the meridians (right).

鍼灸治療の道具はハリだけではない。皮膚を引っ張ることで皮下に刺激を与える吸引治療(写真左)、モグサを経絡上のツボに配置し燃やすことで刺激を与える温熱療法(写真右)も広く行われている

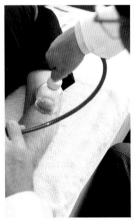

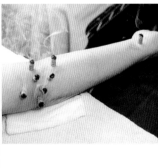

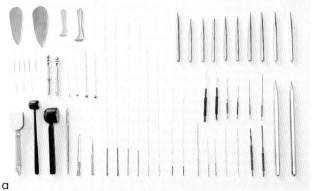
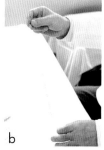
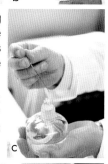

(Image a)Ishihara masters the use of various kinds of needles including kyu-shin ('nine needles') that originated in ancient China as well as those he invented. (b) Needle nearly 30 cm in length (c) The tip of the needle is heated before use (d) Needle for rubbing and scraping (e) Needle made using meteoric iron (f) Needle inserted using a wooden hammer

九鍼と呼ばれる古代中国にルーツを持つ中国鍼から自身で考案した鍼まで著者は多彩な鍼を使いこなす(写真a)。30cm近い長鍼(b)、先端を火であぶって使う鍼(c)、なでる・こするための鍼(d)、隕鉄で作った鍼(e)、木槌で打ち込む鍼(f)

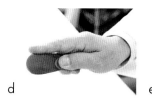
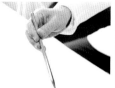
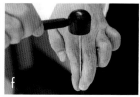

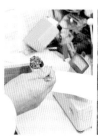
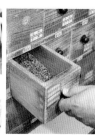
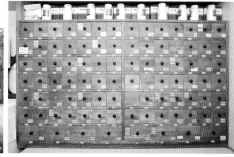

Storage boxes for dry, loose herbs that are the primary ingredients of kampo ('Sino-Japanese traditional medicine'). Dr. Ishihara adjusts the amount and combination of herbs to prepare a blend according to the patient and their symptoms.

漢方薬の原料となる生薬の保管箱(写真右)。生薬の調合は人と症状に合わせ組み合わせや量を変えていく

Fifth Stratum: Divine will level
Universe/Spirit gods(*kami*)

· Unification of physical, emotional, and spiritual awareness
· Behavioral ethics
· Karmic law

· Establishing subjective awareness
· Establishing existential awareness
· Awareness of creative will
· Life-based will

Fourth Stratum: Interactive level
Society/Spirit   Five elements/Earth

· Balance of consciousness and subconsciousness
· Awareness of self-consciousness
· Memory and intuition
· Space-time consciousness

· Water, air, food, plant, animal, other matter
· Weather, topography, climate

Third Stratum: Mind level
Family/Soul

Second Stratum: Emotion level
Others/Emotions

· Emotions and physical balance
· Emotional feedback
· Types of emotions and neurotransmission

· Neurohormones, organs, cells
· Blood circulation
· Immune function
· Meridians

First Stratum: Body level
Individual/Physical body

The Five Strata of the Human Body-field

(See p.63)

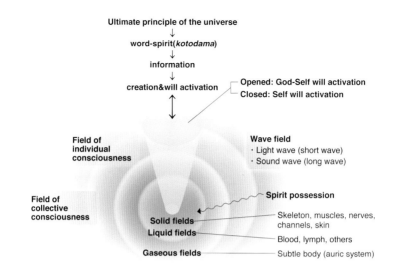

Ultimate principle of the universe
↓
word-spirit(*kotodama*)
↓
information
↓
creation&will activation

Opened: God-Self will activation
Closed: Self will activation

Field of individual consciousness

Wave field
· Light wave (short wave)
· Sound wave (long wave)

Field of collective consciousness

Spirit possession

Solid fields — Skeleton, muscles, nerves, channels, skin
Liquid fields — Blood, lymph, others
Gaseous fields — Subtle body (auric system)

Field of unconsciousness

Human body-field

(See p.60)

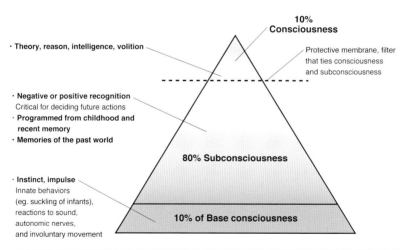

10% Consciousness

· Theory, reason, intelligence, volition

Protective membrane, filter that ties consciousness and subconsciousness

· Negative or positive recognition
Critical for deciding future actions
· Programmed from childhood and recent memory
· Memories of the past world

80% Subconsciousness

· Instinct, impulse
Innate behaviors
(eg. suckling of infants),
reactions to sound,
autonomic nerves,
and involuntary movement

10% of Base consciousness

The Relationship between Consciousness and Subconsciousness

(See p.129)

Illustrated by Hiroshi Kawai

Waki Publishing Corporation
和器出版株式会社

Copyright © Katsumi Ishihara, 2020

Published in Japan by Waki Publishing Corporation
5F Ginza Wing Bldg.1-14-5 Ginza, Chuo-Ku, Tokyo 104-0061, Japan

Author: Katsumi Ishihara
Publisher: Taisei Sato
Translator: Norie Lynn Fukuda-Matsushima
Editor: Kayo Kato, Hiroko Matsubayashi, Kiwako Araya
Contributing editor: Tomoko Takahashi, Saori Kon, Satsuki Takamori,
Yuto Matoba
Photographer: Masafumi Ohana
Book designer: Koji Matsuzawa

ISBN: 978-4-908830-18-1

Printed in Japan by Shinano Book Printing Corporation Ltd.

For further information on
Waki Publishing Corporation, visit our website: http://wakishp.com/

Tel: +81 (0)3-5213-4766
Email: info@wakishp.com

The Mechanism of Life
Illness as Part of Life's Journey

CONTENTS

On the Occasion of the Publication of The Mechanism of Life

Kenji Nanasawa

Director
General Incorporated Association Shirakawa Institute

Modern medicine is hanging by a thread.

At a time when remarkable discoveries are being made in basic medical science, when it comes to cancer, intractable diseases, and influenza, the industry still remains sitting on their hands. I have long pondered as to why this situation has not changed over several decades. What is it that holds back the progress of medical science?

Among the host of physicians and medical experts I am associated with, the person who clearly revealed the answer to my question was Dr. Katsumi Ishihara, a supporter of the study of things Japanese and of *Hakke Shinto* traditions. Dr. Ishihara is a hari-kyu (acupuncture and moxibustion) practitioner who has deified his acupuncture needles with the name 'Kuni no Hari Sonae no Kami' (lit. 'Nation's God of Acupuncture Tools'), and so in that sense he is practicing his techniques with the hand of the kami (the divine or 'spirit gods').

Once I had a sudden intuitive thought that Dr. Ishihara may possibly be the reincarnation of Tanba no Yasuyori (912-995), a historically renowned acupuncturist doctor who played an active part in the Heian era. Yasuyori is famous for editing all thirty volumes of Ishinpo, Japan's oldest medical text that covered and coalesced all of the books on medicine of the Tang dynasty, and was presented to the Imperial Court.

I feel that what is missing in contemporary medical science is not the probing into research of individual cases, but the inclusion and integration of medical knowledge from all fields. In other words, even if one were to be skilled in making close analyses of medical conditions, the concept of integration of general medicine is very shallow. In that regard, the achievements of Yasuyori deserve close attention.

In fact, it was Dr. Ishihara himself who made an attempt similar to Yasuyori. In creating a matrix of phases and hierarchies of every type of medical data, it is certain that Dr. Ishihara's hidden agenda is to change the medical world. That matrix covers a vast scope of treatments, whether used in the east or west, from ancient folk remedies to present day cutting-edge treatments.

From a different angle, this endeavor can be considered to be the integration of the material with the spiritual world—an attempt to see what happens when you combine the information of both and give them a hierarchy; the result is 'The Mechanism of Life,' both the topic and title of this book. And what enabled this result is by no means all craftsmanship-like analogue techniques. As a healing practitioner whose practicum was hands-on, on-site medical care, Dr. Ishihara brought clarity to that world by incorporating science and harnessing digital technology.

In this way, when the Mechanism of Life appears by way of both the tangible and intangible, at last a path to a new epoch opens in medical care. Once the aspects of the Mechanism of Life become clear, it will only be necessary to provide digital measures. Through the above-mentioned matrix, one would easily be able to identify which measures are essential.

What I should draw your attention to are the digital aspects of the Mechanism of Life. The fact that the Golden Ratio can be observed in the alignment of the planets in our solar system signifies that this universe operates like a vast device that is like a dimensional universe computer; and that the 'life' that emerges there can do nothing but obey it.

On a completely different tangent, this past February, our institute established an electronic shrine and succeeded in sending high-quality digitized language data while sending audio and visuals all over the world through the Internet. Through these means, we attempted to trigger a shift in consciousness to its audience. While still in the experimental stages, expected results have already come from those who received the data. At some point, as a part of our collaborative research efforts, I would also like to transmit Dr. Ishihara's matrix of the Mechanism of Life.

It could be said that the weaving looms of ancient Japanese myths have been transformed into today's digital devices. Whether we can bring about an epochal era in medicine depends on our ability to apply digital technology. If expressed in mythological terms, these devices are kami. We have come to an age where humans can no longer evolve without digital devices.

Finally, I thank Dr. Ishihara who has presented the valuable results of his research. I anticipate that this book will deliver the splendor of the Mechanism of Life—a reflection of this vast universe—to the readers who encounter it.

The Mechanism of Life

Illness as Part of Life's Journey

Katsumi Ishihara

Introduction
What is Most Valuable

After working in a particular field for a substantial number of years, one naturally acquires a degree of proficiency and becomes considered an expert or master of that field. I have spent the last 44 years working as a healing practitioner, and since that is my longest term profession, it is only a matter of course that I am often referred to as one. And yet, I have certain reservations about this title.

Despite my sincere endeavors during my tenure as a healer, I am led to question what actual knowledge I have acquired through this work. Often, I question whether I have properly communicated to the world what I have gained as a healer—or more specifically, if I have succeeded in conveying what is most valuable.

Diagnoses and treatments have become more precise, and the numbers of people who have benefitted from my treatments have increased. While these are clear and positive outcomes, they are the natural and ordinary consequence of diligently maintaining a path as a healer.

What I wish to communicate is something else. Its simplicity could be condensed into just a few words, yet such spareness makes me question whether my message would be understood.

With this in mind, I decided I must convey to others what I have long held as my conviction. This is both my obligation as a healer as well as my first stake in the ground along the path I have embarked upon. It was as I arrived at this decision that I was presented with the opportunity to write this book, and all feelings of hesitation transformed into forward action.

I consider all of the patients I have come across along my 44-year journey as a healer to be my teachers, since each of them has graced me with lessons for learning. This multitude of 'teachers' has shaped me and the message I share.

To be sure, while I have shared sincere delight in the progress of those who come to my clinic for treatment, there have been times when results were not always fruitful. Through all of these experiences that have served as opportunities for learning, two fundamental questions that I have sought to answer since my days as a university student consistently resound in my breast: 'What is illness?' and 'Why do people become ill?' I have always held the intuitive conviction that illnesses and their causal relationships cannot be entirely explained through commonly held views of medical care and alternative therapies.

From questions that emerged as I encountered the world of traditional medical care initially as a student arose the inevitable question that I had to confront later as I stood at the actual practice ground. That question is: 'What kind of treatment should I be giving?'

Depending on one's perspective of why people become ill, naturally the notions of ideal treatments also change.

Since my clinic focuses on traditional medicine practices cultivated since ancient times in China and Japan, patients seeking treatment include those who have been rejected as 'incurable' by specialists at the most highly reputed contemporary allopathic treatment clinics in Japan. While each patient's desperate hope for a cure is the same, the cause and conditions of illness for each patient vary, and so I daily face the question of what treatments are appropriate.

So, what happens when such people with 'incurable' illnesses come to me for consultation? There are, in fact, an abundance of instances that would appear to be 'miraculous' to those whose beliefs are limited to contemporary allopathic medical science. It is through these actualities that I am taught and that I gain inspiration. These instances happen not because I have offered treatments particularly unique from others. I implement a variety of modes of treatment that include those that cure with the application of traditional modalities, or adjustment techniques using unseen forces or mind-body approaches that in modern terms may be referred to as 'healing' or 'energy medicine.'

So, what element has supported my work with patients?

Why have I been able to 'miraculously' assist in the recovery of those given up as lost causes by contemporary allopathic medical care? Or, in the case of those diagnosed with terminal illness and a short time left to live, why were they suddenly able to live out their remaining days with calmness and serenity? Considering this question hands-on as a healer, one could say that it is a natural consequence of my experience as a professional, but because fact is more reliable than a dozen theories, this is what I propose:

It is not through miracles that I have made these things possible. It is simply the natural order of things.

In the Meiji period, when Western medical care was introduced on a large scale in Japan, practitioners were taught by Great Britain, the Netherlands, and other European countries such as Germany. However, as I cover in Chapter 2 of this book, the medical approaches of such countries have changed. Instead of using a one-size-fits-all standard to determine which therapies are best, each of these countries has switched to a system that harnesses the favorable points of each treatment. Com paring our medical situation against that of Europe, I think the time has come to review the status quo medical standards of Japan. Of course, in order to make the shift, the general standards of those on the receiving end of the medical treatments must change.

Therefore, upon encountering the ideas presented in this book, I strongly encourage readers to consider today's outlook on medical care and treatment and the bias that exists in viewing treatments based on Western medical science as the only correct form of medical care in the world.

However, this important encouragement is not the most valuable thing I wish to convey in this book.

What I share does not need to be said in a loud voice. It is a plain fact, constantly occurring around us, and lies at the origin of the cause of all illnesses and treatments. It can be summed up in just a few simple words. It is conversely so obvious that we are unable to even see it. Up until now and even today, it is something that has been continually discussed among the most superior authorities in the worlds of medicine and healing. The term that I feel best expresses it is also the title of this book.

That is, 'The Mechanism of Life.'

If you think about it, isn't it fascinating that we have continued to exist here on this planet called earth?

I believe there is a force that has allowed everything to exist since the birth of the universe. It can be likened to the power of the Mother of all life that created the universe and the earth and operates on this globe to sustain our existence as the creatures we call humans—and it is the force that controls the origin of illnesses and healing. No matter how far scientific and medical techniques may progress, it is a force that lies at the origin and cannot be changed. It can be understood as the force that the people of ancient Japan referred to as *kami* (which can be understood in contemporary terms as 'the divine,' or in the animistic sense 'spirit gods'). From our perspective as humans, that force can also be seen as the 'source from which life emerges.' That is why I have named that force the 'Mechanism of Life.'

This Mechanism of Life exists in the foundation of this world and is acting upon all that exists in our world and in the cosmos. While its action gives life to our bodies, when that Mechanism of Life is somehow unable to operate with vitality, it results in a state we call illness. Yet when appropriate measures (or from my perspective, treatments) are given, the process of illness can reverse towards a process of healing.

When the true meaning of the workings of this Mechanism of Life is fully appreciated (or, to use a Japanese expression, 'enters the gut'), or put differently, if illness is firmly understood as another form of one's existence and not as one's enemy, I believe a fundamental change will occur in the relationship between illness and healing, and that will connect to the aforementioned miraculous healing or fulfilling final days of one's life.

What kind of force is this mysterious Mechanism of Life?

Since we can refer to the Mechanism of Life as the law that allows everything that surrounds us in the vast universe to exist, it is not possible to show it, say, on the palm of one's hand. But just as if a tiny ant would try earnestly to understand the body of an enormous elephant, by examining glimpses of the Mechanism of Life that are caught from various angles within processes of illness and healing, we can discover a route for the Mechanism of Life to be able to operate with vitality.

I would like to use this book to establish a dialogue with my readers, in order to present these ideas. What does the Mechanism of Life have to do with illness, healing, and living with vitality in this world? I will endeavor to use all of my experience and learning to bring you an answer to that question.

I

Our Bodies are Microcosms of the Universe

The Daily Mechanism of Life

I-1
Where Did We Come from?

We are inextricably linked to the universe.
I would like to start with a careful contemplation of this concept.

The *material universe is bound together as though it were one, and its various parts are as interdependent as our own vital functions, none of which can be affected without influencing the whole body[...]But there's more to life than mechanics, because these explanations are never complete. They're lacking that one critical element: the life field, the creative force of the universe.*

Robert C. Fulford (2001) *Touch of Life: The Healing Power of the Natural Life Force*

The above excerpt is taken from *Touch of Life:The Healing Power of the Natural Life Force*, a book written by American osteopathic specialist Robert C. Fulford (1905-1997). Since its release over two decades ago, it has become a steady seller in Japan; and I expect a number of my readers will be familiar with it. Dr. Fulford was a medical professional with great experience in conventional Western Medicine. The foreword of Fulford's book was written by Dr. Andrew Weil. A world-renowned leader and pioneer in the field of integrative medicine, Dr. Weil has popularized many medical and health treatments that utilize the power of natural healing, and is well known even in Japan. Weil, who recognizes Fulford as his mentor, is carrying on his legacy by introducing natural health treatments to the rest of the world.

The material universe is bound together as though it were one.

One day, while I was reflecting on how to best explain the Mechanism of Life, this brief and succinct phrase from Dr. Fulford's book caught my eye and I felt the urge to introduce it in my book. In the opening paragraph of his book, he states, '[l]ife cannot be fully explained using the terms of conventional biology, chemistry, or physics.' I imagine that in the United States, where Western medical science is the only discipline to be widely accepted since before the Enlightenment, it must have taken considerable effort for Dr. Fulford's concepts to be recognized. In fact, in the afterword of the Japanese edition, he writes, 'in the US, for a long time I was considered a quack.'

Since medical care is both deeply rooted in and fostered by its surrounding society, there is little chance of expansion into new medical perspectives and practices unless the fundamental ideas of that society change. While practicing as a physician in the US, Dr. Fulford witnessed gradual shifts in societal trends of thought; he said that when he wrote this book, the situation had transformed into one where 'the opinions of maverick doctors became orthodox in medical science,' and 'the majority of American people, who had once turned a blind eye to alternative therapies such as osteopathy, began holding great expectations for them' (excerpt from the translator's afterword). It is clear that the trends of the times had begun to catch up with Dr.

Fulford's way of thinking.

As stated by my esteemed mentors, the times are changing. Regardless of one's whereabouts, the world-view of experienced healers is shifting into alignment. I believe that as long as a medical practitioner or healer is sincerely engaged in treating the bodies of the multitudes who complain of ailments, they are certain to be made aware of the body's autonomous structure—or, as I refer to it, 'the Mechanism of Life'—as articulated by the concept of the 'natural healing force.'

In cases where practitioners may not come to this realization, it is possible that they were misled by clouded perception, or distracted by other issues. The long-standing situation in Japan, however, has been that there are similar circumstances or misunderstandings encountered by the patients themselves, creating an enigma where neither patient nor practitioner can identify what is wrong with the other. Yet once they do become aware, would they be satisfied with the current trends of thinking about illness, treatment, and medical care in Japan? Indeed, merely considering the current situation of inflated medical expenses that threaten the national economy leads to questions.

No matter how affordable various medical treatments become, or how many hospitals are built, and despite the dizzying number of different foods and supplements promising to deliver wellness, the number of people suffering from illness has not diminished at all. I feel that there must be something unnatural about the accepted ways of thinking about illness and treatment. And if there is something unnatural in how we think about illness and its treatment, what is it, and why? I endeavor to touch upon such issues throughout this book.

I came to cherish the idea expressed in Dr. Fulford's short phrase— The universe and man are interconnected as one—and it became the catalyst for my desire to convey the Mechanism of Life to others through this book. To begin, I attempt to trace the origins of our being.

At the birth of the universe, approximately 13.8 billion years ago, an atom sprang from an elementary particle that came from a super string, and joined another atom to form a molecule; and from various arrangements of molecules, matter came into being. In time, the planet we call Earth emerged and life sprung forth, eventually leading to the arrival of humans. These are the ideas described in the current theories of astrophysics and evolutionary science that involve complicated numerical formulas beyond our comprehension, but at the very least, there is one thing of which we can be certain: since the emergence of the universe, it has held its balance through unceasing motion and transformation. Indeed, the universe continues to change and move while gently sustaining a precise order. That is the Mechanism of the Universe.

Life on our Planet Earth, generated within the mechanism of the universe, has an analogous mechanism which also preserves a gentle order in the midst of constant motion and transformation. The various phenomena of life occur in accordance with that mechanism.

For example, when the balance between positive and negative electrical charge in the atmosphere is disrupted, and the potential energy difference between the atmosphere and the earth's surface becomes great, lightning follows with the effect of eliminating the difference. When the balance between the earth's interior and exterior collapses, a phenomenon known as an earthquake occurs. And, as is common knowledge, changes in atmospheric pressure determine the weather; and if there is a vast difference in atmospheric pressure, phenomena we know as tornadoes occur.

Since phenomena such as lightning, earthquakes, and tornadoes possess such colossal energy, they are a menace for us as human beings. From our viewpoint, we would rather not have to deal with these natural events of change. But from the perspective of the planet's harmonic balance, and in the greater scheme of things, these phenomena occur in the natural world for the very purpose of maintaining order in the earth's continually transforming environment.

In other words, lightning, earthquakes, and tornadoes are indispensable occurrences that work to keep a constant order in the earth's environment and maintain a state of balance.

Our bodies, of course, are also included among these natural forces of the earth. The earth emerged in the universe, and we, as humans, emerged on earth. Thus, we can refer to the human body as a microcosmic universe. Perhaps as we follow along this trajectory of thought, various events that occur in the universe which we once thought of as remote and isolated events will gradually start to become familiar.

When we direct our newly opened eyes to our bodies, it is likely we will develop a different perception of the movements of our 'inner universe'; and the idea that disease is similar to natural phenomena, such as thunder and typhoons, may logically arise.

I imagine that the concepts of Dr. Fulford, which I introduced at the beginning of this chapter—'the life field, the creative force of the universe'—will need a little more time until they are discussed with deep accord among the medical community at large. Medical professionals, like other scientists, are faced with the limitations of specialization, inhibited by the narrowness of their single disciplinary focus.

The freedom and generosity we gain by stepping outside the limits of a position or a specialization will be a fine compass for navigating the 'new world.' As a healing practitioner, I would like to continually renew who I am and learn along with others about the Mechanism of Life.

I-2
'Natural Instinct' as One's Innate Healer

An appetite, and a lack thereof.
Both have meaning.
This I learned from my dog who consumed grass
and cured his own illness.

The best approach to study natural instinct is in the observation of wild animals. I learned this long ago from the family dog.

Since this was around my third year of elementary school, it must have been over sixty years ago. Unlike today, in those days most dogs were fed simple meals of miso soup and rice, and in our home it was no different. Dogs, like wolves, are naturally carnivores. Although rice does not suit a dog's constitution, they ate it, as in those days commercial dog food was generally unavailable.

As with humans, when a dog consumes something it is not accustomed to, its body will react in protest. I recall one day we had fed our dog something other than miso and rice—something fatty. Once he ate it, he appeared to lose interest in eating anything else. Concerned, I took him for a walk, and as we approached a grassy roadside he began to eat the grass. Even though he wouldn't touch his regular food, he would eat grass. The following day as well, he ate more grass. Two or three days later, he began to regain a normal appetite.

Even as a child, I recognized that our dog could recover his health naturally from eating grass without any particular intervention. I recall thinking, 'So, this is natural instinct.' Perhaps you have also observed your dog or cat eating grass and been concerned, but in modern terms this is in fact a type of 'detox.' By eating grass, our dog cleaned his gut of the fatty residue that had remained stagnant inside it.

This is how I became interested in observing the behaviors of wild animals. I learned that when they are unwell, wild animals become idle; they rest quietly without eating anything. You might think that unless one eats, one cannot get well. But when food is consumed, the body is forced into the natural process of digestion. And since the body requires energy to work, naturally, energy is needed in order to digest. In fact, it requires considerable energy. And since that need is a significant burden on the body, wild animals have an instinctive understanding of this mechanism. When they are weak they abstain from eating, giving priority to resting the weakened body.

Once an animal is able to move a little, it will first take in water, understanding that hydration takes first priority. After it drinks enough, it will rest again. It repeats this process, waiting until its body has regained vitality. I learned from my family dog that wild animals live by the 'wisdom of living' by their natural instincts.

After years of working in medicine, it became clear that just as there is a reason one's body tells them to eat, there is also significance in one's lack of appetite. It is sometimes necessary for one to eat, and there are also times when one should not eat. Fasting can be beneficial, being an effective way for the body to eliminate toxins and break the habit of overeating. When appropriate, I recommend it to my patients. Moreover, it is also a way to learn through one's own body the significance of abstaining from eating.

I have heard that in the case of some wild animals, such as cheetahs, the hungrier they are, the faster they become. Perhaps you have similarly experienced that your body becomes more agile on an empty stomach. When in a state of hunger, one's vitality becomes explosive. Plants also share this trait. Spring is characterized by a large variation in temperature, and for plants that bud in spring, vitality is enhanced and optimized by this temperature change. While protecting a young life from exposure to cold winds may help it to grow healthy and strong, problems arise once it matures. The organism becomes dependent on protection. This is the same for both humans and plants.

Could it be that our coexistence with animals and plants allows us to learn from day to day how natural instinct and the Mechanism of Life work for our benefit?

I-3
Children Talk with Their Bodies

Children who play outdoors
also toss about in their sleep.
There is a particular reason for this.

The sight of a small child in peaceful slumber is enough to soften anyone's heart. Deep sleep is evidence of an untroubled soul. It is an enviable state for adults with countless concerns about tomorrow and the future, who are plagued by sleepless nights.

With that in mind, I discovered something when observing children at rest: children restlessly toss and turn in their sleep. If one is to compare the sleeping state of an elderly person with that of a child, it is very clear that the older one becomes, the more calmly one sleeps at night. The reason why children are active even in their sleep is likely connected to their youthfulness.

Following this observation even further, I found that children who are active and play outdoors are particularly likely to toss and turn throughout the night. My children (two daughters and one son) were the same when they were little. They slept very deeply at night on the days they spent actively outdoors, and also were the most active in their sleep on those days.

So, what does this mean? Perhaps you will be able to guess based on my observations so far. Restless sleep patterns come from the body's innate knowledge of how to make adjustments to balance out the muscles that have been in active use during the day. Any misalignment or imbalance is realigned while tossing about at night, calming those muscles that were most engaged during the daytime. Thus, the child can run around outside the next day, unaware of his nighttime activity.

By contrast, since elderly people do not move around as actively during the daytime, the misalignment of the muscles is minimal, allowing them to sleep more calmly at night.

This is not a matter of good or bad behavior; rather, it is an outcome of the natural healing process of the body. These responses—turning over in one's sleep to restore the balance of the muscular system, or losing one's appetite when the stomach weakens—are the body's spontaneous process of recovery, yet parents or caretakers are apt to worry about a child's restlessness at night or their loss of appetite.

There is a natural explanation for the lack of an appetite; for example, it may be the delayed effect of late-night dining or snacking the previous night. People eat unnaturally at night, often overeating or 'binging.' This causes excess burden on the stomach, wearing it out. In order to revitalize the stomach, the body reacts by reducing the appetite. When one is experiencing a loss of appetite, it is the body's message:

'Don't eat right now. Your stomach isn't ready yet.' To understand such messages, not just with the head but to let them 'enter the gut,' is the act which we call 'listening to your body.' To do so is to understand the Mechanism of Life.

Listening to the body's message and skipping breakfast is natural, and in fact it goes against nature to ignore that message and force oneself to eat. Through such experiences of listening and healing, one can learn to quit such habits as eating until one is completely stuffed at night or snacking in the middle of the night.

If we believe that our lives are sustained by the Mechanism of Life, the natural healing force that continuously acts upon our bodies, we will naturally notice when we have no appetite or when we run a fever. We will learn to listen to our body's messages in order to figure out the reason behind our fever or loss of appetite. We will find out where the problem is and why the body is reacting the way that it is.

When a child is ill, however, parental affection poses a challenge— we as adults tend to do the opposite of what we should. We take the symptoms too seriously, and hurry to restore the child to his or her former condition. I am sure this scenario sounds all too familiar to parents. Even if the child is not hungry, we force them to eat; we immediately give medicine to lower their temperature. This is the worst way of treating the child when they are ill. By doing so, you are forcibly resisting the power of natural healing that emerges directly from the body.

There is the following case as well: unlike the straightforward issue of overeating or catching a cold, there are times when a child may frequently catch colds or have stomach aches for no apparent reason. If you sense that something is not right, I suggest considering that the child may be communicating something to you. Oftentimes, a child wants more attention from his parents or guardian, and that message is transferred to the body and manifested in symptoms of discomfort.

In fact, this is one of the natural healing forces that a body possesses. Of course, having one's mother notice an illness is the key that leads to healing. Healing becomes simple after an illness is noticed, but noticing is the special power of a mother—the power to receive the message being transmitted by the power of natural healing. I believe that one cannot leave everything up to the body's own natural healing force, but that it takes the power of people and family to harness that force.

I-4
In Praise of Life's Intrinsic Intelligence

**Without our awareness,
our DNA is working in our defense
to counteract viruses and bacteria.
This fact has the power to capture the attention
of even those with suicidal thoughts.**

Within the bodies of all living beings, there are what we call genes that act in various ways to sustain life. Approximately 160 years have passed since the emergence of such scientific theories that suggested such to be the case, and while the first presentation of this hypothesis was said to be presented in 1865 by 'the father of genetics', Johann Gregor Mendel (1822-1884), in what is known as Mendel's Laws, it has since been proven and has become part of common knowledge even of the average person who has absolutely no scientific background.

Yet, even though this has become matter-of-fact, one cannot help but be astonished when one discovers the actual functioning of DNA. Genes are made up of a molecule called DNA (deoxyribonucleic acid), whose structure—as is well known—is in the form of a double helix, and such delicate, ladder-like molecules take action on their own accord to protect our lives, without the need for us to command them to perform this or that task.

The code of viruses and bacteria is firmly embedded in the genetic material that has existed since before the beginning of human life. Also stored is the inherent ability to counteract those very same viruses and bacteria. I refer to this as the 'intelligence' of DNA. For example, when the body is exposed to new viruses and bacteria, this intelligence activates new countermeasures against them, creating new structures by breaking the chain of four amino acids and reconnecting them.

This 'intelligence' can be perceived as the power of adaptation or natural healing, but either way, once enlightened by this knowledge, one cannot help but marvel at the wonders of our human existence. Life forces actively sustain our lives without any conscious effort on our part!

When I speak to patients at my clinic about the Mechanism of Life, some become deeply moved. Among them, there are some with suicidal tendencies, and I sometimes describe in concrete terms the aforementioned genetic activity to reveal to them how our existence—not least of all their own—is being sustained. I suspect that most individuals with suicidal thoughts struggle to endure the 'now,' the present moment. If each moment feels unbearable, the thought of remaining alive for innumerable future moments must eventually become repugnant. Considered from another angle, though, their preoccupation with day-to-day hardships may have clouded their ability to see the preciousness of their existence as a human within the vast universe, supported and protected by the Mechanism of Life.

This is why when I talk about the sustaining forces of DNA, some of my patients who are suicidal are caught off guard and their senses become awakened. They become convinced, deep in their gut, that they are being kept alive by a greater power beyond themselves.

Of course, whether it is learning the life-sustaining power of DNA that resonates, or something that speaks to the soul, depends on the individual. What is important is that one is deeply convinced; a logical, mind-based understanding is not sufficient to promote change in the individual. To hold a conviction of the preciousness of one's existence with a comprehension that transcends thought and logic is deeply significant.

I-5
Cells Think; Skin and Gut Also Have Thoughts

Even though each cell starts out the same,
why does one form an eye,
one an ear, one a brain, or another a bone?
Why do they become as unique as you or me?

Let's open with an example: Say that you are going to build a new home. You decide to have a high-ceilinged living room, a spacious bathroom, and a garden with a lawn. And certainly, the house should have an attractive exterior. Naturally, desire expands to include each wish and whim.

To realize that vision, you will need skilled carpenters. But, even before that, to ensure the desired results, you will need an architect to draft up the plans for the new house. But since each carpenter has their own approach and work style, you should hire a general contractor to oversee the entire construction process and ensure the design is carried out as planned. Ideally, one should have a reliable coordinator with a clear understanding of the completed form of the house to ensure proper results.

Now, what does it take to produce a human body?

Of course, a house is nowhere near as complex as a human body. But like a house, a body is a single composition. Similar to the task of constructing a home, does producing a body also require the equivalents of carpenters and general contractors? A fertilized egg grows into a fetus, which transforms into an infant that is then born into the world; the development from infant to human adult continues steadily over several decades. In that process, 'who' is handing out the instructions?

There certainly exists something equivalent to a drafted plan. As everyone knows, each and every one of our cells contains a genetic blueprint called DNA. The specific instructions for one cell to become part of an eye, another part of a nose, and so on, is encoded in the DNA, which may lead one to believe that it is our DNA that fulfills the coordinator role, or in building terms, the task of the general contractor. But in fact, this is not the case.

Initially, a fertilized egg consists of a single cell. As it develops, this cell—initially a single entity—multiplies through repeated divisions. Yet the DNA in each additional cell is copied from the original cell, and represents the same design plan. Each cell has the potential to carry out any of the instructions of the design plan. In other words, from the outset, every cell has the power to develop into the skin, the heart, or the reproductive organs.

If each cell has the same potential, why does a certain cell become skin, another an internal organ, while others become bones or the brain or the sex organs? Because of the mysterious and complicated phenomenon of cells automatically carrying out different tasks without anyone passing out orders, there was a time when it was thought that the DNA itself transformed as the cells divided. However, approximately half a century ago that theory was debunked through a scientific experiment. It was found that the DNA contained in every cell was the same as the DNA in the fertilized egg.

There are no detailed specifications drafted up in this DNA plan, and there is no one inside your body passing out orders, but nevertheless, a certain cell becomes part of your eye and another becomes part of your nose. While possessing common functions as cells, different traits are also expressed in their final form. This does not happen as a result of a single, accidental chance, but in the natural process of a fertilized egg becoming a human body. In other words, the characteristics of an entire living entity inhabit each cell. To me, this is truly awesome.

For example, consider the eye. The single organ of an eye is composed from a collection of countless cells. The white of the eye and the center of the pupil are each also conglomerations of many cells. Any cell has the potential to become part of the white of the eye or part of the pupil. However, when a certain cell assumes the leading role as the center of the pupil, the adjacent cell takes on the required supporting role, and the cell adjacent to that one is likewise obliged. Each cell acts on its own 'will,' realizing the potential that needs to fulfill its role, and ignoring the potential that it doesn't need, so that all of the cells collaborate to form the organ of the eye in its functional wholeness.

The eye created in this manner connects to the brain through a network of nerves, thereby to perform the function of sight. More specifically, the eye captures light; the retina in the back of the eye converts this light into electrical signals; these electrical signals are conveyed to the visual cortex of the brain where they are decoded; and this information is converted into an image. This mechanism makes possible the phenomenon of sight, or vision. The body can perform the work of seeing only after this complex living network develops automatically.

In the above explanation, I slightly anthropomorphized the cell in saying that it 'acts on its own 'will.'' This phenomenon is described in biological terms as the 'methylation of DNA,' which I learned about in a book by contemporary Japanese biologist Shinichi Fukuoka (1959-). A small chemical substance etches tiny marks on the four kinds of nucleotides that make up DNA; the marks serve to 'switch' a genetic expression on or off, so that for example one cell becomes part of the white of an eye, and another becomes part of a pupil. While this explanation is compelling, I still feel that there are some things that after all cannot be explained from a biological standpoint.

When I say 'the 'will' of the cell,' regardless of whether it is methylation or some other mechanism that creates the physical eye, I think about 'who' turned on this exquisite genetic switch and 'how,' and it helps me consider the existence of some mechanism or force that creates different cells.

If applied more broadly, we are describing the Mechanism of Life, and if limited to the scope of our bodies, we might call it the 'intelligence of life' that resides within the body.

This is easy to understand when considering the act of eating, for example; if you are feeling hungry, when you put something into your mouth, saliva will naturally be produced. If the food chewed in the mouth is carried to the stomach, gastric juices are produced and the food is digested, becoming nutrients that circulate throughout the body. It is not necessary for us to decide to digest food and distribute nutrients. It is the intelligence of life that produces saliva and gastric juices and carries vitamins and amino acids to the places they are needed.

Even in the case where you may be hungry but there is nothing to eat, you do not need to activate your will and intelligence—the natural intelligence of your body voluntarily acts as a coordinator. Producing chemical substances and activating various neurologic modifications, the mechanism that adjusts and sustains the bodily state, after all, exists in the center of our lives.

In recent years, it has been discovered that more than 90% of the body's serotonin—the neurotransmitter known as the 'pleasure hormone'—is made in the small intestine and is connected to the serotonin produced in the brain. This means that just as the brain thinks, the gut also 'thinks.' This is not only true for the gut, but also the skin and heart and other organs, since each is served by an autonomous adjustment function (the intelligence of life) in which each part 'thinks' on its own. In other words, the intelligence of life inhabits every cell of the body.

So next time you feel sick, before heading to a hospital or clinic, I ask that you remember this: your body, with its many networks possessing the intelligence of life, is ceaselessly working to restore itself to a better state.

With that thought alone, perhaps you can improve your understanding of a hospital diagnosis or your attitude towards taking in foreign substances in the form of medication. That small shift in your consciousness will impact your behavior. In other words, it will naturally have a positive effect on your daily life, and that will most definitely be reflected as a positive influence in your body.

II

A Bird's-eye View of Medical Science

Traditional and Allopathic Medicine:
Their Origins and Differences

II-1
Allopathic Medicine and Health

Just as there are things you are capable of, there are things you aren't.
Just as you have talents in some areas, there are areas in which you
don't.
It is the same with medicine.
In Japan, medical care is synonymous with Western medicine.
I think it's about time for a change.

If you were to ask the doctor at the hospital where you are being treated, 'What can I do to improve my health?' what kind of response would you get? Of course, the doctor would come up with a response, but they might be inwardly bothered by such a question, since the answer is outside the specialization of Western medicine.

To most people, medical care is synonymous with Western or allopathic medicine, i.e., the treatment of patients with pharmaceutical drugs and/or surgery to treat or reduce the symptoms of disease. There has been a global effort to adopt Western medical practices, and recently they have become particularly deep-rooted in Japan. Since the Meiji Restoration (1868-1912), Japan has imported a great deal of knowledge from Europe and America. The inclusion of a degree in allopathy in the national qualifications for medical licensing has had a major impact in Japan.

Medical care historically includes many perspectives; there are many traditions of medical treatment around the world, including traditional medical practices and folk medicine in both the East and the West. In fact, the global trend is moving toward a more expansive perception of medical care. Ironically, Europe and the United States—the origins of allopathic medical care—have already adopted a broader and more open-minded approach to medicine than Japan.

For example, since the 1990s medical insurance in the United Kingdom has paid for some of the treatments that are still considered alternative in Japan, and it is rumored that the royal family endorse public support for more holistic practices. It is also well known that Germany, which opened its doors to non-Western medical treatments early on, has established a licensed profession called Heilpraktiker ('healing practitioner'), who can provide alternative therapies without a medical degree. In the United States, interest in alternative medicine has been steadily on the rise, as indicated by osteopathy specialist Dr. Fulford whom I introduced in the previous chapter.

There is no single type of medical care that can cure every ailment. Western medicine is but one of many medical practices found around the world. As a healer with a practice long based in Japanese and Chinese medical traditions, I feel somewhat relieved at the growing recognition of alternative approaches. I believe that at such a turning point, we must come to a better understanding of exactly what Western medical care is. We can make better use of its benefits if we understand the foundation on which Western medicine is established.

IIn that light, we can trace the history of Western medicine back to its origins and arrive at Hippocrates of ancient Greece, who is often said to be the father of Western medicine. Hippocrates (c. 460 - c. 370 BC) is recognized for introducing an empirical approach to the diagnosis and treatment of illness. Before Hippocrates, the dominant Greek view was that illness was caused by unseen supernatural powers. In contrast, Hippocrates developed the theory of 'the four humors' (blood, yellow bile, black bile, and phlegm, i.e. the basic body liquids of the human body) and postulated that illness could be treated by correcting the excess or deficiency of a humor, thus utilizing the natural healing forces of the body. Hippocrates was also known to perform surgery for thoracic empyema (the collection of pus in the pleural cavity). I believe the seeds of Western medicine can be found in his approach.

After Hippocrates, there was little progress until the emergence of a German doctor, Rudolf Ludwig Karl Virchow (1821-1902), who significantly influenced the trajectory of modern Western medicine. Virchow, known as the father of modern pathology, revolutionized the medicine of his era by postulating that 'all cells come from cells,' and in fact this dictum would play an important role in the development of Western medicine.

I believe that Virchow's ideas may have led to the abandonment of interest in the natural healing force at the root of life. It became very easy to trace the cause of a disease: one did not need to consider environment, diet, or the body as a whole, but in the extreme case, only pay attention to the cells. If the cause of an illness is found in the cells, then the cells can be targeted and treated. That which has been found to be unnecessary can be removed, and if viruses or bacteria are wreaking havoc, they can be eliminated. In general, modern Western medicine is the inevitable extension of such ideas.

The premise that all problems are of cellular origin certainly makes it easier to find the cause of an illness or decide how to treat it. In actuality, however, the Mechanism of Life is not so simple.

In a later chapter, I will carefully expand on what elements make up the body, but for now I will simply state that the mechanism that gives life to our bodies is not merely the work of individual cells. The body consists not only of interconnected cells, but also of forces that do not look like cells; for example, there are feelings and thoughts. As an alternative medical practitioner, I am witness almost every day to the adverse effects that thoughts and feelings can have on a cellular level. To be honest, even if I wanted to ignore natural healing forces and focus only on cells as the cause of illness, I could not.

Yet, among medical professionals who have learned from educators who believe modern medical care is synonymous with Western medicine, there are those who hold firmly to ideas that conform to that educational approach. Of course this is not the case across the board, but when I speak of the natural healing forces and the Mechanism of Life explained in this book, which to me are common sense, it is very hard for those who consider Western medicine to be completely authoritative to understand my perspective.

I experienced this while I was treating patients in the metropolitan area of Chiba, before I opened my current practice. I received a complaint from a nearby hospital. In those days I was primarily treating patients with tuberculosis or other serious illnesses with acupuncture and advice for improving certain lifestyle habits. This did not sit well with the hospital and I received an extremely harsh complaint from their representative who said, 'Apparently you are treating a patient with tuberculosis and told them that they will get better. Some nerve!' They even threatened to close down my practice. Since I was not doing anything unethical, I simply responded by saying, 'By all means, be my guest.' But nothing came of it and I continued to treat my patients with tuberculosis, and all of them eventually became well.

If Western medicine is not the one, all-powerful medical tradition, is there another tradition that is? I feel the most effective and globally responsible answer is 'No.' By admitting that there is no all-powerful approach, we can begin a neutral observation of the benefits and limitations of a particular type of medical care. In the case of Western medicine, its primary strength is said to be the symptomatic treatment of patients with acute illnesses, and I agree.

Presently in Japan, when a patient with symptoms of illness visits the hospital for treatment, medical practitioners educated in Western medicine will perform tests to make a prognosis and prescribe medication to control the symptoms, or recommend surgical treatment if necessary. Yet such an approach merely treats the symptoms of an illness, or in other words, they fall into the category of what we call symptomatic treatment.

A clear example is when one is seriously injured in an accident. It is essential to staunch the heavy bleeding and stabilize bodily functions as quickly as possible; acupuncture and moxibustion would be inappropriate. In such a case, there is no doubt that Western medicine, including medication and surgical procedures, is a stronger approach.

On the other hand, when emergency care is complete and the patient's condition becomes stable, a different medical perspective becomes necessary. For example, it would be wise to investigate the patient's core symptoms, and their root causes—in other words, to initiate treatment with a long-term perspective that recognizes the root causes of a disorder and strives for the holistic maintenance of the body. You could say that this is the type of medical care that would directly answer the question posed at the beginning of this section, 'What can I do to improve my health?'

Once we reach this stage of treatment, the approaches of Western medicine that were so beneficial for stabilizing an emergency situation become less useful. This situation, in which a medical approach is more or less useful depending on the conditions, is inevitable. I reaffirm once again the importance of carefully observing the foundations of each type of medical approach to understand when it should be used.

Looking back to my first year as a university student, as I took my first steps to becoming a healer, it is clear that I didn't fully understand what medical care was, much less the true difference between Western medicine and traditional Japanese and Chinese medicine. Thanks to a persuasive invitation from members of the Traditional Chinese Medicine Club on the day of my university entrance ceremony, I became aware of the world of traditional Japanese and Chinese medicine and realized my calling. Rather than becoming distracted by the symptoms of illnesses, I wanted to understand why people became ill. Thus my life as a healing practitioner began.

II-2
My Encounter with Traditional Chinese Medicine

Hives that wouldn't heal even after hospital visits,
And my third invitation to the Traditional Chinese Medicine Club,
Were forks in the road to my destiny…

Destiny is something we recognize in hindsight.

As I mentioned at the end of the last section, I found my path to becoming a healing practitioner after I entered university and encountered Traditional Japanese and Chinese Medicine (or 'TCM' as the latter is commonly known). That encounter provided a current that would carry me toward my fate, if you would call it that. And indeed, it was an enormous current. But upon reflection, there was something that happened earlier that was like a harbinger.

It occurred while I was attending high school. Under the influence of my grandfather and father, who were both university professors, I was pursuing entrance into college to study applied mathematics, but I had failed my first exam and was waiting for another chance to take the exam. Around that time, I ate some mackerel that gave me terrible hives. The mackerel simmered in miso had come from a local fish shop, but it must not have been fresh. Even after several trips to the hospital, the hives would not go away completely. In my search for answers, I read a book on modern pharmacology that explained the mechanism of controlling symptoms with medicine, which I found to be very interesting. So I decided to change my subject of study from mathematics to pharmacology.

Had the mackerel simmered in miso been fresh and had I not suffered from hives, who knows what my fate would have been? Considering who I am today, I believe I would have arrived at this field of discipline no matter what path I took.

After that harbinger, I entered university to pursue pharmacology, and I came across another portent of what was to come: an encounter with the Traditional Chinese Medicine Club (henceforth, 'the TCM Club') at my university. In fact, this, too, did not come out of my own initiative; membership into the club was the result of my inability to turn down multiple, aggressive solicitations from its members.

During university orientation, freshmen are lured in all directions by various university clubs and societies, and while I was visiting the different booths, I was forcefully invited into the TCM Club. Even after I responded that I'd decided to study modern pharmacology, I had to decline a second insistent invitation, and I finally succumbed to the third, telling them I would listen to their pitch. After hearing it, a voice deep inside my gut shouted, 'Yes! This is it!'

I am sure that the pharmacology book I read had interested me, but I think I must have also sensed something unnatural about it.

When I first heard TCM Club members describe the idea that the universe and humans are interconnected, I immediately embraced it. While you may wonder why, I imagine it was because until that moment I had lacked words for what they explained to me.

It may sound like an exaggeration when I say this was my destiny, but I cannot help but think this way when I reflect on my subsequent encounters with various concepts and people of significance, as well as with my esteemed colleague Dr. Kenji Nanasawa who was my catalyst for writing this book.

Since my acceptance of the ideas came so naturally, I am convinced that it was a fateful encounter.

II-3
A New Approach to Perceiving the Human Body

Considering the human body as a system of 'fields' with different properties
Opens up a new worldview of observing the body hierarchically.
Together, let's read and decipher this 'map'
To navigate a journey around the new world.

In Italy in the Middle Ages, Galileo Galilei (1564-1642) rejected the Catholic Church's geocentric model of the universe in favor of the heliocentric (Sun-centered) model, and was subsequently tried for heresy. During the trial he was said to have murmured, 'Eppur si muove' ('And yet [the Earth] moves'). Whether or not Galileo actually spoke those words, history proves that even an authoritarian power great enough to rule the world is unable to establish absolute truth.

Just as the scenery changes slightly when you put on a different pair of glasses, any object that is viewed from a different vantage point will be seen and understood differently. Of course, perceptions of the human body are the same; those who hold that there is only one way of viewing it are generally those with a slightly narrow field of vision.

The familiar signage outside hospital examination rooms is a clear example of how the human body is viewed in Western medicine. The specializations—'internal medicine,' 'surgery,' 'otolaryngology,' 'dermatology,' etc.—clearly reveal an anatomical point of view in which the body is grouped tidily into parts that can be studied independently.

As mentioned earlier, there are strengths in this approach; however, I don't think it can be relied on exclusively. The Mechanism of Life has emerged over an unimaginably vast period of time, 13.8 billion years since the creation of the universe, until we came into being as individual living bodies. In order to completely comprehend the phenomenon of our bodily existence, I have long believed that we need to adopt a much wider and more comprehensive perspective.

It is very natural to consider how the human body interacts in its visible parts—its flesh and bone—and its invisible parts—such as its mind and spirit—and its connections to the universe (such as how the Moon affects the Earth and our bodies). These elements with their varying properties and behaviors become the individual layers that appear to envelop the flesh. I imagine that the body was experienced this way through the exceptional sensitivity of our ancestors. From this awareness, the concept of the human body made up of hierarchical levels, or 'strata'—from that composed of visible flesh to those of unseen energy—has been passed down to the present age.

This view does not perceive the body as only flesh, but rather as an accumulation of layers with different properties. The relationship between illness and healing is naturally reinterpreted when the human body is considered through this filter. Prescribing medication to control pain is a form of crisis management, but this new viewpoint recognizes the need to carefully sift back and forth among the layers in order to discover and treat the root cause of the illness.

These strata of the human body overlap, from the visible physical layers to the layers imperceptible to the naked eye, such as the motions of the mind. While each stratum has its own characteristic properties that function independently, there is also fluctuation that gently opens up to collaboration with other strata. Herein lies the exquisiteness of the living entity generated by the Mechanism of Life.

I now propose that the fields of the human body including its fluctuations can be roughly understood as three overlapping fields of solid, liquid, and gas. I refer to this model as the 'tripartite field,' as shown in the diagram below. While it is merely a simplified hand-drawn conceptual diagram of my personal theory based on the concepts of Chinese and Japanese traditional medicine, it clearly expresses the idea that the body is made up of several fields that overlap in this fashion.

The human body-field can be thought of as multiple overlapping fields surrounding the core of the physical body. Viewed from its exterior, the body would appear as an egg-shaped sphere; a horizontal cross-section would appear as concentric rings, like a slice of a tree trunk as shown in the figure on the right. (See p.55: The human body-fields I)

The tripartite body-field can be divided into two bodies: the visible

〖The human body-fields Ⅰ〗

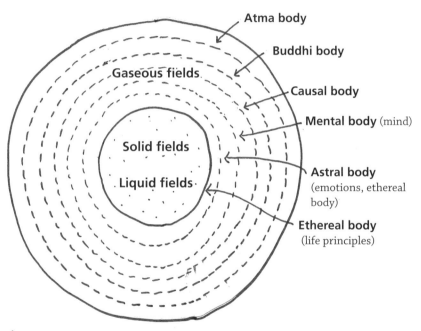

Tripartite Field
- Solid fields: Skeleton, muscles, nerves, channels, skin
- Liquid fields: Blood, lymph, bodily fluids
- Gaseous fields: Ethereal, astral, mental, causal bodies, etc.

body and the invisible body. Conventionally, what we call the human body comprises the visible body (the solid and liquid fields), but this new perspective sees the body as a combination of fields including an invisible body (the gaseous field).

In the diagram, I show an inner circle with a solid boundary line, and several rings with dotted boundary lines around the inner circle. The innermost circle is what is generally referred to as the physical body. In respect to the tripartite body-field, let us assume that this is where the solid and liquid fields are contained.

The solid field is composed of the skeletal body, the muscular body, the neural body, and the epidermal body. The liquids circulating within the body, such as blood, lymph, and other bodily fluids, are closely connected to the solid field and form the liquid field. If disorder, stagnation, or tainting occurs in the liquid field, it also influences the solid field, and manifests as pain, sluggishness, or some other dysfunction. The solid and liquid fields are fused in the human body with close interconnections, and are therefore expressed as one layer in the figure.

Traditional medicines such as acupuncture, moxibustion, and Ayurveda (Indian traditional medicine) were developed in the context of a sophisticated interpretation of the causal relationships between these fields. Each medical approach has its own significance and special characteristics.

The rings that surround the solid and liquid fields comprise the gaseous field. The gaseous field is invisible, but just because it is imperceptible to the naked eye does not mean that it does not exist. I consider this field to have a surprisingly great influence on the modern man and woman who live much more complex lifestyles in much more complicated environments than in the past. Just as the liquid field affects the solid field, changes in the gaseous field influence the liquid and solid fields in many ways. That is why it is important to determine which field holds the root cause of an illness.

According to Theosophy, a European system of thought that emerged in the 1900s, the gaseous field is divided into ethereal, astral, mental, and causal bodies. I will briefly discuss the characteristics of each of these layers.

The ethereal body is the part of the gaseous field closest to the solid field; it is the body in charge of life energy. Harmonizing with the rhythm and waves of other gaseous fields and the universe, it supplies 'qi' ('ki' in Japanese) to the physical body. Qi is the origin of life in traditional Chinese medicine, or the 'prana' of ancient Indian medicine. Because it controls the power of life, the ethereal body is vital to maintaining health and the focus of many traditional medical treatments.

The astral body envelops the ethereal body and is the seat of emotions linked to the mind and extracorporeal consciousness. Feelings can arise from the sufficiency or lack of physical experiences such as pleasure or pain, appetite, or sexual desire; however, there are also sophisticated feelings that arise when humans experience empathetic communities, including sympathy, awe, and affection.

Outside the astral body is the mental body. The mental body is the seat of control of the mind, intelligence, and thoughts.

The causal body envelops the entire gaseous field. It manages the true Self beyond Self. There are various ways to refer to the true Self, including the higher self, the essence of self, the Akashic record, and hyper-consciousness. This body exists beyond the limits of the individual human body, in the sphere of the collective of souls and of hyper-consciousness.

Because the fields of consciousness dissolve into a body of energy or 'Qi,' the gaseous field includes emotions and desire, the senses, thought, and imagination, as well as powers from a higher dimension, such as intellect, love, and soul. Unlike the solid and liquid fields, a great variety of invisible powers gather in the gaseous field, such that it cannot be directly touched or viewed without extrasensory perception. Countless healing techniques have been devised since ancient times to work with the gaseous field. Chinese and Japanese traditional medicine include such techniques, as well as hand healing methods that are employed even today, such as *Qigong* and energy healing, *Reiki*, polarity, and channel *chakra* healing. These therapies deliver healing via the gaseous field of the healer.

By extension, recently scientists have utilized modern technology to invent and develop many devices that act on the gaseous field.(I incorporate into my healing modalities of the *Logostron system* and *Nigi* which has been conceived and developed by Dr. Kenji Nanasawa.)

Now, I would like to share another diagram (See p.60: The human body-field II). This diagram adds new elements to the diagram introduced earlier. Several fields have been added to the outside of the gaseous field. These fields interact harmoniously with the human body-field as a whole, from the solid field to the gaseous field. Furthermore, they are also contact points with the power that forms the structure of the world (universe) expanding outside our bodies. In other words, they are the integration points for the human body-field. You may have guessed that I am referring to the fields of consciousness.

These fields of consciousness include individual consciousness, hyper-consciousness created by groups of individuals, and unconsciousness that falls outside routine, explicit consciousness. Each of these types of consciousness has mutual influence on the others. The state in which one's consciousness is taken over by another was once referred to as 'being possessed,' but this state can actually be understood as the influence of hyper-consciousness or unconsciousness.

The essence of consciousness is greatly influenced by whether it remains at an individual level or opens up and connects to the fundamental principles of the universe, but it can generally be thought of as extending beyond the individual. I imagine those reading this can recall a time when they felt a profound and unexplainable sense of being fully

【The human body-fields Ⅱ 】

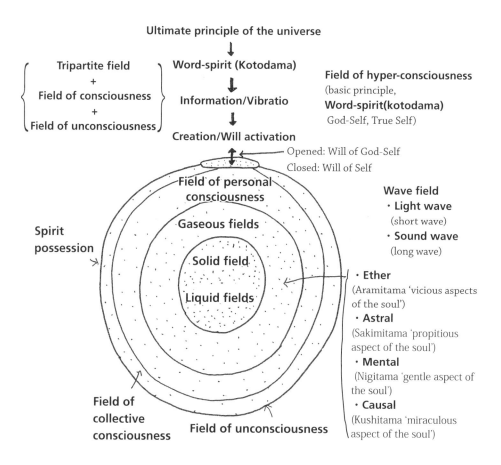

Solid fields, Liquid fields ← Gaseous fields ←Field of consciousness ← Field of unconsciousness

alive beyond their own power and will, and this aroused an intense sense of gratitude within the very depths of the body. That feeling of gratitude is key to accessing the natural healing force that we are born with and continue to possess.

This phenomenon of consciousness and the emergence of a deep sense of gratitude has led to the recovery of many who had received a dire prognosis of illness untreatable with allopathic medicine. In my own practice, I have experienced several instances of healing beyond all common sense. In writing this book, my purpose is to explain that to learn about the Mechanism of Life is to connect to the fundamental principles of the cosmos and the fields of consciousness.

The various contemporary methods of psychotherapy, hypnotherapy, the introspection method, and others are ways to access a person's field of unconsciousness. Changing the field of unconsciousness is also connected to bringing out one's innate potential to heal naturally.

I learned fairly recently that this superior model of the human body as a multilayered entity connected with the cosmos has existed in Japan since ancient times. It impressed me greatly when Dr. Kenji Nanasawa taught me about *Hakke Shinto*, a branch of *Shinto*, the animist tradition of Japan that can trace its legacy back more than 10,000 years. Hakke Shinto was preserved and handed down by the *Shirakawa* family which controlled the religious services of the Emperor in ancient times.

I became aware of Hakke Shinto at a very opportune time, thanks to the wise decision of Dr. Nanasawa—the equivalent of a modern day schoolmaster of Hakke Shinto—to make public the teachings of its ancient wisdom. In those teachings, the fields, from solid to gaseous and including the fields of consciousness, are wonderfully expressed in a five-layered concept as divine will level(kami), interactive level(rei), mind level(kon), emotional level(jo) and body level(tai). It can be surmised that this concept must have arrived from the physical sensations and insights of our ancestors without the use of analytic scientific techniques.

If one were to compare the five strata of Hakke Shinto (See p.63: The human body-fields III) with the illustration shown previously, 'the body' would be the fusion of gaseous fields and the fields of consciousness from emotions to kami with the solid and liquid fields of an individual. The functions of the emotional and mind strata can be inferred from the words themselves, but to me, the interactive, or spirit, stratum refers to the fields of consciousness that link person to person, society to individual, and individual to kami.

At the very top of the hierarchy is the kami stratum. Although the word 'kami' (or any equivalent such as 'divine,' 'higher power,' or 'source') may conjure a religious or supernatural association, in fact, as mentioned above, it signifies the field of consciousness that connects to the foundational principles of the universe, opening up beyond a personal level.

When the fields of consciousness remain stuck at a personal level,

【The human body-fields Ⅲ 】

Ultimate principle of the universe

↓

Word-spirit (*Kotodama*)

Sympathetic vibration, → ↓ ← Information, vibration
resonance

Creative will activation

gods of heaven
(*Amatsukami*)
gods of the land
(*Kunitsukami*)

‖←Membrane→ Opened: Will of God-Self
Closed: Will of Self

Five Strata

五階層(Gokaiso)

Divine will level
神(Kami)

Interactive level
霊(Rei)

Mind level
魂(Kon)

Emotion level
情(Jo)

Body lebel
体(Tai)

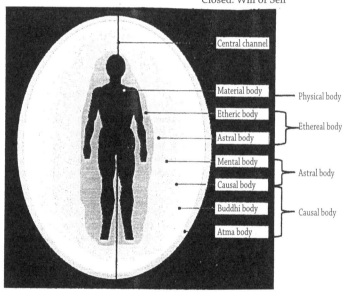

Central channel

Material body — Physical body

Etheric body
Astral body ‑ Ethereal body

Mental body ‑ Astral body
Causal body

Buddhi body ‑ Causal body
Atma body

The Human Energy Field

Adapted from *Vibration Medicine* (2001) by Richard Gerber

the will of Self is exercised; when they open up beyond the level of the individual, the foundational principle of the universe and Self become one, exercising the will of the God-Self. In order to explain the implications of this, I added some explanatory notes to the diagram; rather than understanding these concepts with your mind, it is important to naturally find resonance (although it has been used already in this book several times, I prefer the phrase 'gut feeling').

This map of the five strata of the human body-field is a superior concept to help refine and apply one's modalities as a healer. I would like to convey this message to as many people as possible through this book. While it may extend superfluously beyond the topic of healing, I encourage anyone with deeper interest to attend Dr. Nanasawa's lectures or read his books.

As we observe the human body in its multiple layers, I believe that everyone will start to naturally grasp the true potential of holding a variety of viewpoints in medical science. With several decades of work as a healing practitioner under my belt, I say this with sincere conviction: medical care that focuses only on the solid and liquid fields of the human body cannot appreciate the essence of why we suffer from disease.

II-4
Harnessing the Body-Field Perspective in Treatment

Each of the human fields has a role and is interrelated with the others. This understanding naturally affects the approach to treatment. One will also be able to know precisely which field to treat.

For those who now understand the concept of a human body-field but not how to use it in their treatments, I would like to simply explain field relationships from the perspective of a healer.

I will start with the relationship between the liquid field and the solid field.

There are many examples of successfully treating symptoms rooted in the solid field by directly treating the solid field. In traditional Eastern medicine, treatment modalities include massage, shiatsu, acupuncture, moxibustion, and chiropractics, all of which rely on the forces of natural healing. As in the case mentioned earlier, if one has a deep physical injury and is heavily bleeding, hemostasis is the most urgent priority; in that case, the most responsive practical solution is surgery based on Western medicine care. Since treating the solid field puts a halt to a worsening body condition, for the time being emergency treatment will end here.

There are other examples where symptoms such as pain are observed in the solid field, but solely treating that field is ineffective. If the healer were aware of the relationships within the body-field, they might determine that the root cause was in the liquid field, which includes bodily fluids such as blood and lymph. It may be that a tumor has formed or that viruses or bacteria have spread due to an impure or imbalanced liquid field. This is an indirect approach.

Accordingly, the solution would be to purify the liquid field. If its balance is optimal, the spreading viruses or bacteria would disappear and the body's dysfunctions would revert to normal. This illustrates the reason for treating the liquid field.

There are many methods for adjusting the liquid field, including traditional medical therapies such as homeopathy, traditional Chinese medicine, Ayurveda, thalassotherapy (seawater therapy), and blood-letting. These traditional approaches harness the powers of natural healing to treat the liquid field. If the body's condition returns to normal after eliminating abnormalities in the liquid field, the rest will be taken care of by the body's innate healing power, and the body will usually return naturally to an optimal state.

The gaseous field can influence both the liquid and solid fields. Understanding those relationships gives rise to ideas about using the gaseous field to restore the liquid and solid fields. Healing methods for the gaseous field include Qigong, acupuncture, moxibustion, *Chi* therapies, hand healing, Reiki, and wave therapy using machines (for example, the Logostron system, *Takada Ion*, *AWG*, and the *Metatron bioresonance machine*).

These three fields—the solid field, the liquid field, and the gaseous field—can be thought of as mutually affecting each other while each possessing its own identifiable characteristics. The challenge in healing the body-field is determining which field should take precedence over the other. Emergency situations in particular require a precise judgment of which field should be treated first.

In such circumstances, a specialist who thoroughly understands the tripartite body-field of solid, liquid, and gas is an ideal judge, since they can precisely determine where to begin treatment by observing the condition of the entire body-field. In some cases, the patient will have abnormalities in the liquid field, yet the moment requires immediate attention to the solid field.

Practitioners who target only one of the fields make all decisions based on that narrow frame of vision and consider treatment focused only on that field to be sufficient. However, those who comprehensively understand the tripartite body-field are familiar with the roles of each field, and are thus able to discern, for example, the futility of trying to treat one field before treating another; for example, they sense when treating the gaseous field would be premature and focus instead on adjusting the liquid field. Yet, those whose entire practice is exclusively based on a singular approach tend to insist on treating only one specific field.

In other words, the most important thing is to understand the role of each field and how it interacts with the other fields; this allows the healing practitioner to harness the power of the fields to the utmost. Such insight should be expected of all those involved in medical care, conventional or alternative alike.

Now I will introduce the fourth field: the individual consciousness. This is a vital field that affects all of the other fields. In fact, the field of individual consciousness is fused with the gaseous field. The functions of emotions and spirit expressed in the gaseous field can also be understood as the effects of consciousness, subconsciousness, and hyper-consciousness. In that sense, a wide range of invisible subfields occurs in the field of consciousness.

The field of consciousness has three subfields: individual conscious-ness, hyper-consciousness, and unconsciousness. Because each of these can affect the solid, liquid, and gaseous fields, when any part of the field of consciousness becomes disturbed, so do the solid, liquid, and gaseous fields.

So human consciousness intervenes in all of the fields: consciousness influences thought, thought influences emotions, and the tripartite body-field manifests the influence of consciousness. This is a critical point that I would like my readers to keep in mind. This implies that by changing the emotional and mental elements of consciousness, or by changing any other elements of consciousness, you can also change the tripartite body-field.

Certainly, if the solid field is too badly damaged, emergency medical treatment may be necessary. Although there are ways to repair the solid field by changing the field of consciousness, when there is limited time one may need to give priority to the solid field while modifying the consciousness. This is a case that tests the healer's depth of understanding of the human body-field.

According to the Hakke concept of five strata of the human body that I introduced earlier, three of the base strata—body, emotion, and mind—are affected by self-consciousness. This would imply that the physical body, emotions, and mental state of a person can be altered by changing self-consciousness. With the higher fourth and fifth strata of the body-field, on the other hand, the energy of the 'God-Self' (the connection to kami, the principal source of the universe) becomes most important.

While the 'Self' that belongs to the tripartite body-field can be changed by altering one's consciousness or subconsciousness, the collective body beyond the tripartite body-field (which could be called the 'public' body-field) can only be changed through the power of the fields beyond consciousness and subconsciousness. I will save the details of this concept for a future opportunity.

II-5
The Function of the Chakras (Force-Centers)

**The connection between the visible body
and the invisible body.
An invisible pipe-like connection
assumes that role.
The people of old called these 'chakras.'**

To recap, the bodies of human beings are made up of two bodies: the visible body (the solid and liquid fields) and the invisible body (the gaseous field). Long ago, in any part of the world, this is likely how a majority of people conceived the body, at least until the spread of modern science. Earlier, I introduced the perspective of European Theosophy; now, I will introduce the ideas of ancient Japan by way of the animistic tradition, *Shintoism*, in which these ideas are incorporated. In Shintoism, the human body is separated into containing the physical, ethereal, and astral bodies. It can thus be said that the perception of death as the end of the physical body's activity is only a recent idea.

Considering the traditional view of the human body, one obvious question arises: if the body consists of visible and invisible bodies, how are the two bodies connected?

There may be an invisible pipe-like connection between the visible and invisible bodies. This concept was probably found all over the world at one point, but the people of ancient India named the connection 'chakra,' meaning 'circle' or 'wheel' in Sanskrit. Those who practice yoga are very familiar with this term.

Metaphorically, the chakra can be compared to a bypass connecting the visible bodies (the solid and liquid fields) and the invisible bodies (the gaseous field, or in terms of Theosophy, the ethereal body, astral body, mental body, and so on). For example, if negative thoughts emerge from the body that controls mental activity, they are transmitted through the chakras to the astral body, which is one layer beneath. Since the astral body is a gaseous field that controls emotions, stress resulting from negative thoughts influences the intensity of the feelings, and there is a stagnation of pent-up feelings.

Furthermore, when stagnant feelings are transmitted from the astral body through the chakras to the ethereal body that controls the life energy ('prana'), and then to the physical body, a functional disorder also occurs there. If the functional disorder continues at length, eventually a negative chain reaction will result in a mechanical disorder

In this manner, the chakras connect the fields of the body-field. There are several different theories regarding the number of chakras. For example, among 'New Age' theories, the navel is not considered a chakra, but in Theosophy, Indian yoga, and Tibetan medicine, it is. In Tibetan Buddhism, it is thought that there are five chakras, including the navel.

The importance of the navel is clear when you consider that a pregnant woman is connected to her unborn child's navel via an umbilical cord. Thus, in my practice, even when my patients have trouble in the third chakra (the solar plexus), if I strongly sense a problem with the navel, I approach treatment from that direction.

Since contemporary healers are primarily influenced by New Age theories, I will describe the characteristics of each chakra according to that perspective.

The diagram (See p.73: The seven Chakras) shows the frontal chakras of the body. Seven chakras are aligned around the body's central canal (the 'Sushumna') that runs along the spine.

The first chakra is called the Muladhara, or root chakra, and is located at the perineum. In the female body, this is between the anus and genitals, and in the male body, it is near the base of the spinal column. Since it is the chakra closest to the earth, it is closely related to one's way of connecting or uniting with the earth. Those with strong first chakras are grounded in their thinking and have a firm connection with the earth. On the contrary, when the first chakra is closed or unstable, one is unable to think in a grounded way, and their thoughts tend to float adrift. An imbalance tends to manifest physically in the area around the genitals or anus, close to the first chakra.

The surface of the second chakra is the 'tanden' (abdomen) or Svadhisthana, the inner part of the lower abdomen just beneath the

〔The Seven Chakras〕

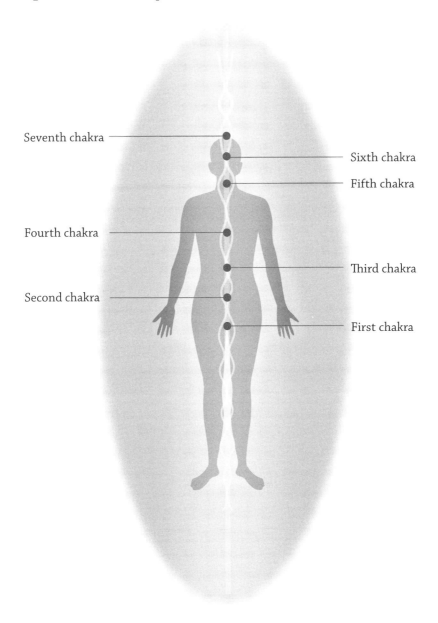

navel. The rear side, just behind the abdomen, has two chakras fore and aft; these are called the sacral chakras. In general, the anterior chakra is related to emotions and the posterior chakra to volition. The tanden contains the 'tsubo,' or acupuncture meridian points) called 'Kikai' and 'Kangen,' both 'Conception Vessel meridians'). Because the tanden is where life energy (prana) is controlled, a stable second chakra means the force of one's life energy is very powerful. This is why martial artists train so intensively to strengthen the tanden. Therefore, when the second chakra is at full potential, one is full of vigor. When it is lacking, one is easily worn out and the legs become weak.

The first chakra is red and the second chakra is orange. The small intestine is highly susceptible to emotions due to its close connection to the second chakra. There is a tendency for the intestines to become hypersensitive, causing diarrhea at the moment something unpleasant occurs in social situations.

The front of the third chakra, or Manipura, is located just below the pit of the stomach. It is the chakra most deeply related to the digestive system.Its color is yellow, and it is based in the solar plexus. This chakra reveals the strength that a person has in their self-consciousness; when the senses of accomplishment, self-esteem, and ambitions are high, this chakra opens and it functions at its highest level. When one holds back from doing what one wants to do and acquiesces to the whims of others, the chakra will be closed, and diseases of the digestive system may appear.

The front of the fourth chakra (Anahata) is the heart. Its color is green. It influences the cardiovascular rather than the respiratory system, and it is also related to the thymus. This chakra is referred to as the 'love chakra,' as it controls love. When this chakra is activated, the energy of love flows easily, but when it is irregular, one's self-centered behavior dominates. If there is someone you know whose every action appears ego-centric, it is possible that they have a closed fourth chakra. It is difficult for those who didn't receive enough affection from their parents as children to activate this chakra. Thus, this chakra's functioning is related to a person's upbringing and environment as a youth.

The front of the fifth chakra (Vishuddhi) is the throat. Its primary color is blue. Verbal expression is the problem most associated with the throat. If one is able to express their feelings and thoughts in a candid manner, this chakra is steadily activated. If one suppresses one's feelings for fear of harming or upsetting others, the throat chakra will naturally become clogged. When a reserved person tries to suppress their anger, the red energy of anger may be exposed as a sore throat.

The front of the sixth chakra (Agnya) is the third eye. Its principal color is indigo blue. The third eye is the chakra connected to the power of intuition. Despite its seeming importance for healing, there is no longer any focus on training about this chakra even in traditional medical practices such as acupuncture and moxibustion; only palm readers still train this chakra. Palm reading was extremely popular in Japan from the Taisho era to the early Showa era (c. early 1910s to1930s). Palm readers would examine the negative aspects of their customers by intuition, moving their hands over their bodies to discover what part was under duress. Since it was believed they could not become healers without such a skill, they made considerable effort to train the third eye.

When the third eye is trained, even beginners show strong intuition, and they are assumed to have the potential to become good healing practitioners. The power to foresee and clearly capture the essence of something at a glance is enabled through the third eye. When this chakra is closed, one is reluctant to use intuition to understand the material world, quantum physics, or the world beyond the five senses. If this chakra is opened, however, there is a danger that conceit or overconfidence will lead to a connection with the world of the dead, so self-reflection is advised.

The seventh chakra (Sahasrara) is located in a single spot at the crown of the head. Its color may be purple or white. Like the sixth chakra, it is related to the pineal or pituitary gland. As the first chakra controls one's connection with the earth, the seventh chakra controls one's connection with the heavens. This is the place of exchange between the heavens and humans, and when this chakra is opened, one can smoothly enter into the spiritual world or the higher realm of the gods. On the other hand, those for whom this chakra is closed tend to think that the physical world is the only world and cannot extend their consciousness beyond it. This chakra contains the love of the Universe and the power to integrate the Universe with the Self, making this chakra the most significant among the seven chakras.

II-6
Comparing Chinese and Japanese Traditional Medical Science–Ideological Views of 'Qi'

Kamiho, the medicine of the divine; waho, traditional Japanese medicine; and *kampo*, Japanese medicine based on traditional Chinese medicine–
Starting with these three medical approaches, Japanese traditional medicine has developed into a unique practice grounded in Japanese culture and thought.
By exploring traditional medicine in China, the roots of kampo,
Let us observe the characteristics of Japanese and Chinese traditional medicine.

When it comes to Japanese and Chinese traditional medicine, most people first think of kampo, otherwise known in most parts of the world as 'Chinese traditional medicine,' or 'TCM.' Naturally, this leads to the question of whether kampo is the traditional medicine of Japan or whether it originated in China. Since the Japanese word kampo uses the Chinese ideographic characters 漢 (kan, or 'China') and 方 (ho, or 'way'), it is natural to assume that kampo is the equivalent of the traditional medicine of China.

The interpretation of kan is correct, but it is more natural to assume that kampo refers to medicine developed in Japan based on Chinese medicine. Over 1,600 years have passed since TCM reached Japan from across the sea. Despite their shared origin, the concepts and methods of

Japanese and Chinese traditional medicine evolved in different cultures and historical contexts. So, the key question is: What are the similarities and differences between Japanese and Chinese traditional medicine? To gain perspective on this interesting subject, let us briefly unravel the history of medical science in Japan.

We will start first with a look at ancient Japanese medicine.

Tracing the history through old documents about ancient Japan, such as Kojiki ('An Account of Ancient Matters') (c. 712), Nihon Shoki ('The Chronicles of Japan') (c. 720), and the Kogo Shui ('Collection of Ancient Stories') (c. 807), we learn about such approaches as incantations of various kami (or 'spirit gods')to treat illnesses, herbals remedies for both humans and animals, and the use of stone needles (for bloodletting). Since these practices are clearly distinct from the traditional medicine that developed in China, they can be considered to be indigenous ancient medicines of Japan. To invoke the sense of original medicine, I call it the 'way of the kami' medicine. (In the past, the character 方 [ho], or 'way' in English, was specific to medicine, and it was used to describe the most specialized techniques used in a particular medical approach.)

Although such ancient indigenous medical approaches have not received much attention in the present age, it is worth knowing that prior to the eighth century, Japan had a form of medical care which, although not fully systematized, was based on unique perspectives of medicine and life.

On the other hand, systematized medicine that emerged and developed in China also reached Japan at about the same time. What is now known as acupuncture, moxibustion, and traditional Chinese medicine (TCM) were apparently introduced to Japan during the reign of Emperor Ingyo (412-453), along with Buddhist medicine. These approaches soon entered mainstream Japanese medicine. When the Taiho Code was enacted in the year 701, establishing administrative and penal codes in the Confucian system of Tang China, Chinese medicine found its place in the national system.

The 19th article of the Taiho Code regulates medical and pharmaceutical science. Starting with the appointment of medical instructors, the Code defined specialties for students of pharmaceutical medicine, study methods, and precautionary measures for preparing medicine for the Emperor. The Code also stipulated the years of professional study required in each branch of medicine: for example, internal medicine required seven years; pediatrics and surgery each required five; ears, eyes, and oral care, four; acupuncture, seven; shiatsu (acupressure), three; and exorcism through spell incantation, three.

At the beginning of the Heian era, acupuncture doctors became established within the system alongside other medical experts. In addition, under imperial command of Emperor Heizei, documentation of local medical treatments was gathered from various parts of Japan, and this was compiled into a 100-volume encyclopedia, the Daido Ruiju Ho, which was published in 808.

Since original manuscripts of the Daido Ruiju Ho do not exist, there is no way to know how much has been altered throughout history. Nevertheless, it is often referred to as Japan's oldest medical text. I consider these medical remedies and practices collected from various parts of Japan to be the Japanese counterpart to the Chinese traditional medicine that has been handed down since ancient times.

As I will mention later in this chapter, it was during this era that acupuncture physician Tanba no Yasuyori completed a medical text called Ishinpo, which was presented to the Imperial Court in 984. This is, in fact, Japan's oldest intact medical text.

It is unclear whether traditional Chinese medicine, as it was systematically understood in Japan, was referred to as kampo, as it is not recorded in the Taiho Code or other literature prior to the Heian era. The term 'kampo' does appear in documents dating to the Muromachi era (c. 1336-1573). It is also clear that from the Edo period (c. 1603-1868) onward, kampo became widely known and practiced.

Today, kampo generally refers to the medicine primarily made from plants, but historically its definition extended beyond medicine to include acupuncture and moxibustion therapy. For example, in the Edo era, kampo was used to describe medicines in the form of decoctions, pills, and powders. Decoctions were prepared by boiling medicinal herbs in water. For the most part, kampo referred to the use of such medicine for medical treatment. After the Edo period, as society changed with the times, kampo specialists increasingly incorporated acupuncture and moxibustion in their practices, and kampo became more closely associated with these modalities.

In any case, kampo has become one of Japan's traditional medical sciences through the development and evolution of a medical tradition that originated in China.

Over time, the three trends of 'kamiho' (medicine of the kami/divine), 'waho' (traditional Japanese medicine), and kampo (traditional Japanese medicine based on Chinese medicine) have influenced one another, with kampo (including acupuncture and moxibustion) taking the central role in a framework of Japanese traditional medicine.

And then there is China. The traditional medicine of China, the precursor of Japanese traditional medicine, is called Chu-igaku ('Chinese medicine') for short. In addition to acupuncture and moxibustion therapy, treatment with decocted medicinal herbs is also based on Chinese medicine, and so evidently the basic therapies of Japan and China share some similarities. However, I believe that historical circumstances in Japan and China led to differences in the philosophical foundations on which their medical practices are based.

The appearances of plants and crops vary depending on the soil in which they grow. In the same way, the traditional medicine that originated in China took root in the soil (i.e. thought) of Japanese culture and eventually became unique to Japan. Such changes are natural, and there is no point in trying to establish which is better or worse. But since the differences of thought on which a medical science is based are significant, I will touch upon them here.

All matter of the universe is composed of a vital, material force called 'ki' (more commonly, 'Qi'); this view, called 'qi monism,' is common to both Japanese and Chinese traditional medicine The main point of qi monism is that Qi is the origin of all matter in the universe, which means that there is some kind of constantly transforming life source.

When the density of Qi is light, it has no form. There are various things that exist but do not have form, like sound and wind, like heat and cold, like the human soul and feelings that are not visible but have an effect. Like these, there is an appearance of energy in the body that we call 'qi.'

When Qi becomes dense and heavy, it takes on a form that can be seen and touched. In the process of taking form, the concrete matter of Qi becomes differentiated, emerges, and transforms. This concept is key to understanding qi monism.

The understanding of Qi may be the biggest difference between kampo and Chinese medicine; Qi can be perceived to have the monism of the T'ai chi, the 'Grand Ultimate,' or it can be perceived to have the conflicting cosmic dualism of Yin and Yang. It is my belief that this is the main diverging point in the approaches of kampo and traditional Chinese medicine.

In kampo, Qi is a singularity; in other words, it can be considered as 'one.' In the practice of divination in Japan, the T'ai chi, or 'Grand Ultimate,' also is the 'Oneness' that is an undifferentiated absolute and infinite potential that is ever-present in a world of unity. The same is true of Qi in kampo. The Qi in T'ai chi sometimes has a Yin aspect and sometimes a Yang aspect, but both aspects share the same original Qi. In terms of the body, the state of illness and the state of health both are expressions of a source Qi, and at the root, they are the same; this is the conceptual approach in kampo.

On the other hand, a holistic understanding of Chinese medicine, from which kampo originated, touches on such concepts as the Tenjin Goitsu, or 'Unity of Heaven and Man,' and in terms of the two original sources of Yin and Yang, this is significant. For stable, optimal health, the balance of Yin and Yang must be even; various phenomena will occur if the balance is upset. If illness emerges, it is understood that there is a clash between the vitality of Yang and the malevolency of Yin. If vitality wins out, an illness can be cured, but if malevolency is stronger, the illness will progress. In that case, how does one suppress malevolency and how does one strengthen vitality? If one thinks of Yin and Yang as opposing forces, then it is natural to think along these lines.

Of course, the philosophy of 'Oneness' also existed in ancient China. If one were to unravel the ideas contained in the Huainan-zi ('The Writings of the Huainan Masters'); the Lei-zi (the third of the Chinese philosophical texts in the line of thought represented by the Laozi and the Zhuang-zi, and the writings that describe and encapsulate Daoist philosophy); and the Daodejing, one can observe the lively unfolding of the philosophy of 'Oneness' in such theories as San Cai, or three interconnected natural forces of the universe, earth, and humanity, and Tian-ren-he-yi, or the idea of the unity of the universe and humanity, as well as others that discuss the integral approach of man and nature and the universe.

What changed this trend of monistic thought was the emergence of Neo-Confucianism in the Song Dynasty. In Neo-Confucianism, Qi constitutes the world and is the basis of existence, and 'Li,' or reason, provides the law. In the resulting Li-Qi dualism, Li and Qi depend on each other to create structures of nature and matter. When the Theory of Li-Qi is later applied to humans, it is understood as a dualism of Qi (dispositional nature) and Li (inherent nature), reversing the theory of 'Oneness.'

Influenced by Neo-Confucianism, the theories of Chinese traditional medicine also began to shift from the unified dualism of ancient Chinese medicine to the dualism that inhabits modern Chinese medicine. If Yin and Yang are considered as two independent sources, the idea of opposition and unification inevitably follows. Compare this to the unified dualistic view, where Yin and Yang emerge from a single source, and you can see the similarities.

If seiki ('spirit energy'), or the power of resistance, conquers jaki ('evil energy'), then vitality is restored. But if jaki wins out, illness will worsen and lead to death. It is a battle between seiki, or 'correct, anti-pathogenic' Qi, (life force) and jaki, or 'evil, pathogenic'.

Qi (harmful forces). This is the basic premise that ties the ancient thought of Chinese medicine to that of the present age. While a correlation with the Western medical approach may seem unlikely given the difference in culture, if you reinterpret the singular original source Qi as two opposing forces of 'sei' (anti-pathogenic) and 'ja' (pathogenic), the result will be understood anywhere in the world.

There is a fundamental difference between the theory that there are good and bad Qi (seiki and jaki), and the theory that they are integral parts of a whole. In kampo, Qi is a single element, and seiki and jaki are integral, and so the appearance of healing forces that are generated from one Qi is considered a symptom; the support of that symptom is called treatment. Techniques and treatments are needed to assist the good energy and eliminate the bad when supporting healing forces.

That there is such a fundamental theoretical difference between Chinese traditional medicine and kampo may be attributed to the religious and philosophical backdrop—during the Edo period (1603-1868) in Japan, many kampo doctors were Zen Buddhist priests. On the other hand, in China, those learned in Taoism were involved with traditional medical treatment, but Zen priests did not have any active role as doctors.

Those who study traditional medicine and become practitioners without exposure to the background philosophy—how easy is it for them to learn the treatments for combating bad energies and supporting good energies when symptoms arise?

I personally believe that how the brain developed in response to linguistic differences also affected the divergence of Japanese and Chinese traditional medicine. It is well known that although they are both Asian languages, Chinese grammar is closer to the grammar of European languages, including English, than it is to Japanese grammar. Furthermore, many other attributes of the post-Neo-Confucianism era may have also affected the divergence of Chinese traditional medicine and Japanese kampo.

That is as far as I will discuss the differences between traditional Japanese and Chinese medicine. Next we will focus on acupuncture, which is used as a modality for treatment in both medicines.[1]

II-7
Acupuncture—Taking Tradition to the Future

In the past, acupuncture needles were used as scalpel-like tools for surgical treatments,
As well as for healing illnesses.
These needles became streamlined into a form
That could be used for any acupuncture treatment
Here I reveal the story of old and new acupuncture
Including its history with such fateful breaks from tradition.

Acupuncture and moxibustion (the burning of moxa, or dried mugwort on acupuncture points, or 'meridians') are two treatment methods that are representative of traditional Chinese and Japanese medical therapies collectively known as 'hari-kyu.' They date back more than 2,000 years to ancient China.

There is a set of acupuncture needles called kyu-shin, or 'nine needles,' which were used in China in ancient times. This set contained nine different types of needles, whose shapes and usages have been passed on to the modern age. However, there are presently very few acupuncturists in either China or Japan who are skilled in their application.

When I tell other hari-kyu specialists that I use kyu-shin, they are invariably surprised because the needles are not common for practical use. But this set of needles shows the variety of tools that were used for acupuncture long ago. They come in a number of shapes and sizes, from thick to thin and long to short.

The variety of needles was probably due to the circumstances of medical care at the time. There were no scalpels available for surgical procedures; many illnesses had to be treated externally with needles. As a matter of necessity, needles were designed for a variety of purposes: needles for healing by touch and by scraping, long needles for penetration deep beneath the skin, needles for stabbing for bloodletting, and so on. The diversity of shapes and lengths suggests that a wide range of medical therapies could be handled through acupuncture treatment.

The hari-kyu techniques of ancient China were propagated to ancient Japan by way of the Korean Peninsula. Ishinpo, which we described in the previous section as Japan's oldest intact medical work, was written two years into the Eikan era during the Heian period (984), and its 30 volumes are now preserved as national treasures in the Tokyo National Museum collection. It describes medical practices that are said to have originated in the Sui and Tang Dynasties, and also details the key acupuncture points and treatment methods of hari-kyu. The author, Tanba no Yasuyori, was a court physician occupying the rank of 'acupuncturist' that had been established under the Taiho Code.

Subsequently, physicians of kampo and 'waho' (native Japanese medicine) embraced acupuncture, and it became a mainstream modality of healing from the Muromachi period to the Edo period (c. 1336-1868).

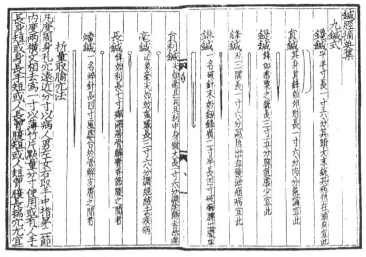

The oldest existing *kyu-shin* images
Reprinted from *Zhen Jing Zhai Ying Ji* (1965) by Du Si Jing

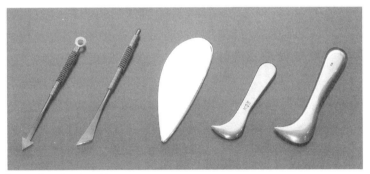

Forms of *zanshin, kyu-shin*
Reprinted from *Visual de Wakaru Kyu-shin Jitsugi Kaisetsu* [Nine Needles Techniques in Visual] (2012) by Tokyo Kyu-shin Kenkyukai [Tokyo Kyu-shin Research Society]

During this timeframe, when the country was relatively closed to outside influences, a uniquely Japanese acupuncture technique emerged. In the 16th century, a Zen Buddhist monk named Misono Mubunsai (1559-1616) discovered a needle technique, 'uchibari,' that could adjust the internal organ by tapping a long needle with a mallet to dispel jaki (noxious/pathogenic qi) and gather seiki (correct/anti-pathogenic qi).

Another technique was discovered by a blind acupuncturist, Waichi Sugiyama (1614-1694), who served as the physician of Shogun (military ruler) Tsunayoshi Tokugawa (1646-1709). Sugiyama is credited with devising a method of using guide tubes, pipes shorter than the needles, to help guide the needle vertically into the patient's skin. This insertion technique is still widely practiced in Japan.

The acupuncture needles used by hari-kyu specialists today are based on the needles used in the Edo period. Some acupuncturists still use the 'enri-shin' (round-sharp needle) or the 'sanryo-shin' (three-edged needle used in bloodletting), and many of the narrow needles formerly used by blind acupuncturists are still used for the guide tube insertion technique.

There have also been improvements that made the narrow needles introduced from China even narrower, and the development of several needle shapes for scraping the skin. Other than these, there have not been any significant developments worth mentioning in a uniquely Japanese acupuncture.

In fact, I can't hide my disappointment with the degeneration of techniques and approaches to an almost primitive state of acupuncture, in comparison to an age when needles like the ancient kyu-shin could be used to treat almost any medical situation.

As Japan steadily trended toward the ubiquitous application of a uniform type of narrow needle, China somehow maintained its use of diversely shaped needles. Not that every acupuncturist was able to use all nine of the kyu-shin needles, but at the very least, a practitioner could select their tools of trade—be it long needles, heated needles, or narrow needles, reflecting their approach and character. Regrettably, however, the Chinese tradition was wiped out in a single stroke during the Cultural Revolution.

While there had been a shift to general-application needles used strictly for insertion, ultimately the most defining influence was the Cultural Revolution. In this chaotic age, a majority of Qigong masters and influential acupuncturists were killed; those who were not murdered fled to Taiwan.

It would be misleading to state that there were no notable practitioners of traditional medicine left after the Cultural Revolution. However, the truth is that the once-thriving field of traditional acupuncture became stunted after the watershed of the Cultural Revolution. The so-called academics who taught university students did not have much skill as practitioners, but they came to occupy most of the clinics, and the selection of needles changed. The narrow needles in China are thicker than the common needles used in Japan, but practitioners have increasingly used only narrow needles instead of a variety of needles.

There are only a few acupuncture masters remaining who are as proficient as the late Dr. He Puren (1926-2015), Chinese founder of the Santong method ('three methods to remove stagnation of Qi'), which is now widely used in China for over 100 clinical applications. Dr. He was known for his mastery of a variety of methods—most significantly his Santong method, which is a combination of manipulated needling methods of go-shin (filiform needling with solid needles), ka-shin ('fire-needle' therapy, or 'red-hot' needling), and sanryo-shin (or 'triple-edged' needle for blood-letting). Sadly, Chinese acupuncturists who can skillfully use all nine of the kyu-shin needles have all but disappeared. And, unfortunately, only the logic and the dialectical theories of kampo have been adopted.[2]

Despite my introduction to the unfortunate unraveling in the history of acupuncture, I am also able to report on its brighter prospects. In hopes of reviving the use of kyu-shin in practical applications of acupuncture, an acquaintance gathered a group of interested persons in 2005 to pursue the potential of hari-kyu beyond current styles and schools of practice. It is called the 'Tokyo Kyu-shin Kenkyu-kai' (Tokyo Kyu-shin Research Group). In spite of my limitations, I serve as the group's chairperson with the intent to inform practitioners and students of the possibilities for kyu-shin.[3]

It may seem that we are attempting to discover the new by scrutiniz-ing the past, but we are also undertaking a new, unprecedented exploration. One avenue is the study of materials for making acupuncture needles. Iron has been used as a material for needles since ancient times, and later, in the Momoyama era (1568-1615), an acupuncturist in Kyoto named Misono Isai produced needles of gold and silver. Today, needles are generally made of stainless steel, but in fact, the effect of acupuncture treatment varies depending on what material is used.

For example, gold is a powerful metal that attracts Qi. Because gold is an extremely foreign metal to the body, it is my hypothesis that the body deploys Qi in an effort to eliminate the needle from the body. On the contrary, platinum is familiar to the body and can be thought of as having a high affinity with the body.

Whether my hypothesis is wrong or right, I believe we can achieve a more precise treatment effect through the successful exploitation of the relationship of certain needle materials and their impact on the body. In considering new materials for acupuncture needles, when I heard Dr. Kenji Nanasawa's aforementioned proposal to use iron meteorite and silicon for acupuncture materials, I felt inspired.

As is well-known, the iron meteorite is made of iron and nickel, also known as meteoric iron. It is a precious metal with a limited supply. Dr. Nanasawa commissioned an experienced master-swordsmith to produce a sword using meteorite iron, an undertaking I was able to observe, but I am ignorant as to whether any needles have been made from this alloy. Acupuncture needles made of meteoric iron would be a historic first. What kind of action and effect would meteoric iron, a metal delivered to the earth from outer space, introduce as acupuncture tools? For that matter, silicon with a purity of more than 99% is used in acupuncture, and it has the highest affinity with the human body.

Dr. Nanasawa continues to encourage me with new ideas, such as the potential of using the mineral agate. Although it was not my natural inclination to use minerals as material for acupuncture tools, I have been inspired and encouraged to take up the challenge.

Amid such a whirlwind of ideas, a single idea from traditional medical practices can open up a world of potential, and I have been moved to the realization that there is an unknown world awaiting us.

The freshness of taking lessons from the past every day—could it be that traditional medicine is indispensable and inseparable simply because it is traditional medicine?

Note

1 Concerning the structure of the brain, I referenced Nihonjin no No ('The Brain of the Japanese') by Tadanobu Tsunoda. It goes into detail about the function of the brain and Eastern and Western culture.

2 Developed in 1984, a 'small needle scalpel' therapy by Dr. Hanzhang Zhu was a ground-breaking invention, sparking a second revolution in acupuncture. The application of his small needle scalpel therapy is still rapidly expanding.

3 For anyone who is interested, please refer to the website and feel free to join my lectures.

III

The Voice of Illness

A Message from the Body

III-1
Where Does Stress Come from?

**Stress is the same as illness and wellness.
It builds up because one imagines the existence
of something nonexistent,
Once this is understood,
one will suddenly become aware of many things.**

There is a well-known Japanese expression, 'If you take a closer look at the ghost, you will find only withered silver grass,' meaning that if fear overpowers your emotions, even the ears of silver grass appear to be ghosts. This illustrates a common phenomenon: careful observation of a situation reveals that it is not what it appears to be at first glance. This is also true for many situations in contemporary medicine that I have touched upon in previous chapters of this book.

As I mentioned in a previous section on the theory behind kampo (Japanese medicine based on traditional Chinese medicine), *Qi*, the 'life force' at the origin that gives birth to all life forms, can be thought of as one world of the T'ai chi (the 'Great Ultimate'). In Japanese tradition medical care, illness and health are manifest in the different appearances of that entity. I find the best definition for that 'one' world to be 'the Mechanism of Life.' In any case, once this perspective is adopted one should easily be able to accept the idea that both illness and health are one and the same. That is to say, to begin with, there is no such thing as either illness or health.

When I tell my patients that the same applies to the so-called 'stress' that seems to affect everyone in the modern world, most of them will shake their heads and say, 'Doctor, you are wrong. I am definitely suffering from stress'; but the truth is that there is merely a condition of the body that is perceived as 'stress.'

For example, those who sense something unpleasant in their physical condition and interpret it as 'stress' may assume that as long as they take the weekend to indulge in their favorite pastime, be it hiking, sports, or whatever, they can rid themselves of this 'stress'; and once it is released, they can face work on Monday with a renewed spirit. Yet, by the time Friday comes around, they find that stress has accumulated once again, and so they repeat the stress-releasing weekend activities in order to make it through another workweek. While this positive release of energy may be healthy, it is not a sustainable solution. Such repetition has to end at some point; fundamentally, the accumulated stress does not truly disappear.

In fact, when one experiences something as stress, you need to focus on the origin of that sensation. There is something in particular that is making a person feel the stress, and unless that problem is settled, the perception of stress will return again and again. It is critical to ask oneself why that situation is stressful, and unless one pins down the exact problem, there can be no lasting solution.

Imagine the following scenario: While at the office, from out of nowhere a co-worker says something that hurts your feelings. In response to their words, you might find yourself on the verge of conflict. But then you recall what kind of person that co-worker is ordinarily, and their typical day-to-day behavior. Once you realize that what they said was out of character, you may naturally wonder what influenced their unusual behavior. If you ask them if anything is wrong, they may respond by telling you about some trouble they had at home that morning, or maybe that they are irritated because of all their overtime hours and lack of sleep, or some other response that would give a clearer picture.

Once you hear your co-worker's explanation, the sense of discomfort that you felt at first should immediately fade away. On the other hand, if you take their hurtful words at face value, you are sure to be left with unresolved feelings about what occurred.

Similarly, you may be able to understand why stress is not something that will simply go away after some 'stress relieving' activity. The real problem lies with the root cause of the so-called 'stress.' Instead of trying to eliminate something that doesn't exist, it is essential to focus on the foundation of what is actually troubling you.

This is what I mean when I say that stress is a matter of perception, and in fact, does not really exist. Everyone experiences some kind of sensation when things do not go as planned or when something unpleasant occurs. Some won't let themselves react and won't allow that experience to be converted into stress—they repress their feelings behind a veil of reason. I will talk about the danger of this habit in a later section.

To summarize, when a person experiences some kind of frustration, and chalks it up to stress, and decides the best thing to do is to release it through exercise or play, they will invariably run into the same situation over and over. On the other hand, if people try to locate the origin of their sense of unease despite the difficulties, they should be able to arrive at a basic solution that can resolve the problem altogether.

The same holds true for the process of entering true healing from a state of illness. What is the basic cause that produces a poor health condition? If earnest attention is paid when confronting the illness, a particular cause can certainly be found.

Those who realize that their bodies are telling them to take a close look at their lifestyles or ways of thinking and make positive adjustments have in fact already begun the process of healing. I often say, 'Illness is a message,' and what I mean by this is that illnesses are messages from the Mechanism of Life.

In the next section, I will discuss messages that illnesses send us.

III-2
Anger and Stomatitis

Was it something spicy I ate?
Or could it have been a lack of sleep?
That might be the case, but there also may be something more.
What can be learned from this small mouth disease called stomatitis?
Let's think about it.

Whether I'm treating a patient or presenting a lecture, I never miss an opportunity to tell people this: being ill is not something to entirely reject; illnesses contain messages from the Mechanism of Life. If you can receive and accept those messages, your life will be enriched.

Yet many people who are only familiar with general hospital treatment are convinced that illness is just something to eradicate— when the symptoms are gone, that's the end of it. Although they may not be immediately receptive to my words, they may start to listen and respond if they don't see any improvement with hospital treatment.

When I talk about this, I often use examples of different illnesses to illustrate my point—to show what kind of messages can be received from a particular illness. For instance: stomatitis, or inflammation of the mucous membranes of the mouth or lip, such as canker sores.

Stomatitis is a common condition that is probably experienced by most people at some point in their lives. If you sense some kind of irritation either on your lips or inside your mouth, it is most often a sign of stomatitis. When it progresses, even a touch of the tongue can cause sharp pain, and it gets harder to enjoy your meals. In that sense, it can be a troublesome condition, but it rarely becomes severe and typically gradually goes away. Once the pain is gone, as is human nature, you will immediately forget that you had been so inconvenienced by it.

Of course it is understandable to think the condition is healed once the pain is gone. However, if you dig a little deeper into the underlying problem, you might be surprised to uncover the true cause, opening up an entirely new state of awareness.

I have learned from my own clinical experiences that inflammation inside or around the mouth is a message from the body. This is true not only for the mouth—each part of the body has a role to play in sending messages.

These roles depend on the innate force within one's body (the force I refer to as the Mechanism of Life or the Network of Life), which is not only physical, but also cooperates with the other layers, such as feelings and will. When the work of the Mechanism of Life is inhibited for some reason, the body will sense that and try to restore it to its normal function. This is what I have referred to several times as the natural healing force and, once it is exercised, it manifests as pain or heat or some other symptom of the so-called illness. The symptoms inform us that something in the body is out of order and that the body is working towards recovery. These symptoms such as pain and fever are just one example of what I call 'messages from the body.'

Now then, why do symptoms such as pain and heat appear on the inside and periphery of the mouth? In the case of stomatitis, this is the key point; why the mouth and not the ear or nose? The answer lies in its relation to the function of the mouth as a part of the body. Think about it: what kind of work does the mouth do?

When the mouth functions properly, it is the entry point for air and food and the exit point for exhaling and speaking. However, when stomatitis occurs, those properly working functions become hindered. If one experiences pain each time one eats or talks and something touches the inflamed area, anyone would become close-mouthed. And so with this as a hint, what could the relation be?

For example, let's imagine that something happens that you can't accept. You become resistant and want to deny how it is affecting you. Perhaps if you recall a specific situation with a family member or friend, you will understand what I'm talking about. In such situations, what generally lies at the root of your emotion is anger. Since you are aware that the situation will become awkward if you openly reveal your anger, you instead choose to remain silent. But still, there is no way to resolve the anger that remains inside you. Although the angry words rise in your throat, you swallow them instead.

If you continue to suppress your anger for too long, your body will find other ways to do the work of expressing it. If not through words or actions, the work will be done some other way. This is a natural process.

The stomach is one of the locations where this work is done. For example, unsettled feelings of concern or disagreement may lead to a loss of appetite. In terms of the human bodies discussed earlier, suppression of feelings occurs in the fourth body, or the mental body. Next, the suppressed emotions appear in the third (astral) body, where sensations and emotions occur, and affect the stomach and intestines of the first (physical) body. Just as we talked about with stress, a symptomatic treatment such as gastrointestinal medication will restore the appetite only temporarily. What is at the root is the repressed emotion. Where does such a feeling of repression arise? Once you find the answer to that question, you should be able to see true signs of recovery.

So then, what happens when one represses an even fiercer emotion like anger? In that case, it is often the mouth, not the stomach that is affected. Ideally one should transform anger into the energy of words and spew them out, but because they can't, the energy of anger collects and is stored in the mouth. Then, since anger is expressed as heat, it erupts as inflammation in the mouth. It is only a matter of time before it will progress to stomatitis.

Of course, stomatitis has more causes than one. Since inflammation is a product of the activity of healing power working to disperse the accumulation of heat inside the body, stomatitis may break out if one eats something spicy. In this case, because it is a physical problem of the first stratum of the human body, the symptoms will naturally dissipate if one abstains from spicy foods for a while.

But if a person who does not generally enjoy spicy food should all of a sudden have a craving for it, they should suspect that there is a specific reason behind that craving. Sometimes a person will consume more spicy food than usual to try to blow off the pent up steam of dissatisfaction or other unresolved emotions. The stomatitis may in fact be telling you to be conscious of the reasons behind your craving.

The same is true for allergies. Repressed feelings are located at the Origin, and they manifest as some disorder of the body. But often the messages that illnesses are trying to convey is that there is a problem that has not been sensed in one's day-to-day awareness. Illness may be similar to owning a smart pet dog: when the master is about to cross a dangerous bridge, an illness takes the lead and becomes alert to the danger. Instead of using words, illness uses the power of pain or fever as a warning. If people become aware of this aspect of illnesses, the view that they are only something to escape or avoid will gradually start to change.

III-3
Why Ears Stop Hearing

A sudden loss of hearing,
or an unexplained leg pain that makes it harder to walk
Medical examinations don't reveal the cause...
For such times as well,
it is best to start by listening to the 'voice' of illness.

Once in a while, I receive visits from patients with sudden concerns about hearing loss. They want to know if they are becoming hard of hearing. Their hearing had been normal up until a certain point in time, and then it suddenly became hard to hear. If not related to congenital impairment or aging, the first suspicion would be sudden sensorineural ('inner ear') hearing loss (SSHL), commonly known as sudden deafness. In this case, I believe that the same conclusion would be drawn by doctors of Western medicine and traditional medical practitioners. This would also be my first guess.

A sudden loss of hearing would be upsetting to anyone. It's understandable why most of these patients ask whether they can be cured, since the impairment would affect their work and daily life. Because there may be some with the same concern among the readers of this book, I will first divulge my prognosis: While the time for healing may vary from patient to patient, there is no need for concern. The condition is certain to improve.

Now, here is the story I want to tell:

As I mentioned in the previous section of this chapter, illnesses always have a message; most likely, sudden deafness has an important one. What could be the message it is trying to convey? Let us speculate.

For example, let's say you visit a general hospital and ask the doctor what could be the cause of your sudden deafness.

If I were a doctor of Western medicine, I might be slightly at a loss for words. This is because in contemporary Western medicine, the cause is not yet known. You may be surprised that even in an age of advanced research, Western medicine still cannot explain the cause of sudden deafness. But if one were to investigate the many circuits that deliver sound from the ear to the brain, it would not be possible to find a concrete defect. That the cause of this condition is evasive is one of its characteristics, and so a doctor's explanation will depend on their particular theoretical approach.

On the other hand, if the doctor's range of knowledge extends beyond medical science, they may investigate the cause by listening to the patient's history and the circumstances surrounding their hearing loss. However, such doctors are few and far between in today's Japan. In most cases, you will be prescribed medication and asked to return for more observation. As an emergency measure, that is one means of treatment, but it leaves the question of the true cause of the hearing loss unanswered. And while the underlying problem remains, naturally there is the possibility of relapse.

This is why it is important to earnestly consider the message that the condition is trying to teach you. One extremely helpful tool going forward is the perspective of the fields of the human body taught me by Dr. Kenji Nanasawa, which I have discussed previously. Although the symptom of SSHL—'suddenly becoming hard of hearing'—is a condition occurring at a physical level, the absence of a detectable physical problem suggests the influence of problems in other strata. If that is the case, where does that leave us? After repeated explorations of that question, I came upon the understanding of the origin of SSHL and have been able to clarify my theory.

Imagine that the ears are transmitting the message that it is easier not to listen. Then the supposition can be made that the sound one is hearing is the actual problem.

When I asked if there was any troubling matter in their lives prior to their hearing problems, one patient recalled, 'Come to think of it, I wasn't getting along with my boss at work and even his voice started to grate on me. Before I knew it, my hearing had worsened.' It was easy to deduce that since the mere sound of his boss's voice, the patient didn't want to hear. It's as simple as that.

The body is honest. The emotional stratum sent the message that the boss's voice was unpleasant, the mind stratum sent the message that it did not want to hear that voice, and the attentive ear complied by shutting down its hearing function. You could say that the network of life collaborates to realize the wish of the patient—in this case transforming the mechanisms of the body to make it harder to hear the voice of his boss. Since that change occured on more than just a physical level, no matter how much testing is done through the Western medical approach, it should be obvious that the cause of the hearing deficiency cannot be found.

Since there is basically nothing wrong with the patient on a physical level, if they were to become aware of the root cause of the ailment and make a conscious effort to resolve it, the ear would heed that intention and follow suit. A proactive decision on the part of the patient to listen to their boss's words and all other sounds will, in effect, set them on the road to recovery. In fact, once the patient turns their attention from their anxiety about their hearing loss to the underlying cause of their deafness, it is like a bright ray of light penetrating through a dark tunnel, and it is not unusual for their condition to start improving without much more effort.

Of course, there are other illnesses besides hearing loss that are sparked by the negative feelings that arise in human relationships.

Once there was a patient who one week earlier had suddenly lost his ability to walk and had to be carried into my clinic by his parents. He was about 30 years old. Up until then, he had been able to walk normally without any trouble, but he was suddenly affected by pain in his hip joint and knees and had to take time off from work because he could not walk. Since it was not the result of any accident, the cause was a mystery. He wanted to know what could be done.

In fact, I already knew the cause when this patient came to my clinic; but since it was not proper protocol to call it out immediately, I first treated him lightly with acupuncture and then turned the conversation to his work situation.

As I expected, his job seemed to be demanding. Although his contract hours were from eight in the morning to six at night, in actuality he left his house at six a.m. every day and didn't return until after midnight. He had been brooding over whether he should consult with his boss about his working conditions, but didn't want to risk being fired since his wife and children relied on his income.

The origin of the problem was similar to that of the patient who developed sudden hearing loss due to a negative reaction to his boss's voice. The latter patient's legs cooperated with his feelings of not wanting to go to work where he had been subjected to severe demands. Since the originating cause of the patient's condition could not be treated solely with acupuncture, I focused on the patient's feelings, and offered to negotiate with his boss if he was unable to do it on his own.

With such an encouraging offer, he became determined to take charge of the situation on his own. After consulting with his boss, he was able to restore the initial terms of the contract, and was subsequently able to return to work after only a week.

Even if his health had improved on its own, if the harsh demands of his job were not resolved, any decision to return to work would have retriggered his feelings of apprehension in the third stratum of his body, and he would have run the risk of relapse.

This case impresses upon us the truly well-designed nature of the body. A man who could not walk and had to be carried into my clinic by his parents restored his ability to walk after only a week, by altering his feelings to become positive and taking action to change his situation.

At the same time, this was a remarkable example of the amazing accuracy of the messages conveyed by illness.

III-4
Cancer is a Questioning of One's Lifestyle

**Observing patients with cancer
living out their lives with verve
makes me think:
Perhaps cancer is an illness that possesses power—
a power that influences a forward-thinking action.**

Anyone who unexpectedly encounters painful situations may at some point ask themselves: 'Why do I have to go through such pain? Was it something I did?' When the challenge is an illness-even more so when it is cancer-the diagnosis alone is enough to drive a person into the depths of depression.

There are also those who ask me: 'Doctor, you say that illnesses always have meaning, and that they have messages toward that end. If that's the case, does it mean that the cause of the illness is within oneself and it is one's own fault?'

Perhaps for them, this way of thinking is hard to swallow. It may be better for me to simply give an ambiguous reply such as, 'No. There are multiple causes for illnesses.' But on the other hand, I know very well that this would only ease their mind temporarily. Indeed, a careful choice of words and direct communication will have better results. Holding this conviction in my heart, I respond to them earnestly as follows:

'It may be hard for you to accept at first, but instead of placing blame on others or on bad luck, the better approach is to imagine that this illness is trying to convey a message to you. It is telling you to take a good look at your lifestyle and make changes. With this perspective, one day you will find yourself thanking your illness.'

I once had a visit from a patient who had an operation to surgically remove one breast due to breast cancer. She had been taking chemo-therapy drugs after the operation, but after half a year, her condition worsened again. Cancer had been found in her liver, and the hospital gave her more medication, but when she sensed it was not improving, she came to see me through the introduction of an acquaintance.

When I first talked with this patient on the phone, I asked her what she wanted me to do for her and she responded, 'I want to learn how to live.' This meant that she wanted to distance herself from the approach of surgical or medical treatments and instead review her lifestyle and make proper adjustments.

And so, when she came to my clinic and told her story, she spoke endlessly of the pent-up resentment she held against her mother-in-law. Apparently, ever since her marriage, she had been tormented by her. And so I suggested, 'Why don't you purge yourself of all the negative emotions related to your mother-in-law? I would like you to write down all your feelings of dissatisfaction and anger.' And when I added, 'You could even write, 'I wish she were dead,'' she said, 'Okay, I will.' And so she wrote down every last thought about her mother-in-law.

You may think that your negative feelings can be banished by conscious reasoning, but in fact they are firmly rooted in the subconscious. Instead, if you write down your negative feelings and release them in concrete form, they will naturally fade away. Once you write down every last one of your negative feelings, a sense of composure will return and your thoughts will be much clearer.

After some time, I asked the patient, 'So, how do you feel about your mother-in-law now?' She responded: 'I realize now that she was lonely like me. I can now see that somehow her only means of surviving was to torment me. Once I realized how sad she was, I could not stop my tears from flowing...'

The spite that had driven her to murderous thoughts before venting her antagonism had completely changed, transforming into an empathetic desire to do something for her lonesome mother-in-law. I later heard that astonishingly, the once harsh mother-in-law became amenable to the patient's efforts and became kind to her, rousing thoughts of the synchronicity that analytical psychologist Carl Jung spoke of.

I had the patient come in for a visit after three weeks. If she still had had lesions, ordinarily I would have detected some blockage during the examination; but as I did not, I told her that it was likely that the cancer was gone. And sure enough, test results brought the good news that, as

I had expected, the cancer had disappeared.

I was thrilled. I told her, 'I'm so pleased for you. Through your cancer, you found the divine.' She responded that long before she learned she had cancer, she had become a Christian to help save her from her emotional struggles. However, she seemed to realize that what had actually saved her was not some external God, but her own power—which is what I meant by finding the divine-and she decided to abandon her religious pursuits.

This patient, by releasing all of her hatred and grudges against her mother-in-law, instantly eradicated the selfish feelings brought about by the sphere of her ego. Then, as if claiming her own feelings, she realized that her mother-in-law was also suffering from loneliness and sorrow, and she transformed her anger into empathic tears-I think it was at this moment that the power of healing emerged.

There are other times when I was taught in various ways by my cancer patients.

Observing patients whose cancer disappeared, like the one I just talked about, as well as those whose cancer remained but who carried on their lives with vigor, I often felt that a great shift in consciousness had occurred. They didn't remain in despair after getting cancer, losing hope in their future. Rather, it appeared that owing to their cancer, each patient gained a greater state of awareness.

Of course, as described above, with any illness there comes an awakening. For example, in the case of a cold, we are made more aware of our daily lives. A fever makes us wonder if our unnatural lifestyles make our blood impure and the fevers help to eliminate impurities through the power of natural healing. This kind of awareness becomes an opportunity to make us review our eating habits and lifestyles.

Yet since ordinary colds are not generally a matter of life and death, the level of awareness remains relatively shallow. In the case of cancer, however, despite the increased chance of recovery, it is still a potentially fatal illness even in the present age. The gravity of cancer means that it can convey profound messages related to the origin of life; in a sense, I believe this is the role of cancer.

Well then, just what is this deep message about life's origin that cancer conveys? Put succinctly, I would say it is this:

I believe that the urgent message cancer gives us is to awaken to the realization of how one's life is sustained and supported. Despite being aware of our faults, under ordinary circumstances we don't set out to change them. The impact from a mere cold may stir our intent to improve our lifestyle, but it is not grave enough to move us beyond that point. Unless you are a raging optimist, however, a cancer diagnosis will rouse thoughts of mortality. To think about death is to reflect on one's life and to consider how to live out what remains of it.

You may begin to question whether you have been leading a good life and whether you should continue as you are. When sought in earnest, the answers you find are sure to be uniquely yours. Your thoughts may become flooded with memories—perhaps of a friend with whom you had unresolved issues, making you realize in fact that their role was to fulfill the unsavory task of reminding you of your inner struggles. You may have naively felt that you alone were responsible for your survival, but now you awaken to profound gratitude for the forces of life that you have been granted.

Such thoughts that begin to well up passionately from the depths of one's being are immediately transformative. This is because such consciousness is connected to the deep root of life itself. From that moment onward, the Mechanism of Life starts to demonstrate its power to heal.

So, at every opportunity, I tell people that cancer is not something to fear, but a precious voice from inside that you were formerly unaware of; and the patient becomes transformed once they recognize this.

For my patient who had concerns about her mother-in-law, the instant she let go of her hatred for her and became filled with gratitude, it became less of an issue whether or not she had cancer. In the end, it was the patient herself who banished her cancer through her change in attitude, and she felt a natural sense of gratitude for the cancer cells within her. Feelings of gratitude do not come from a person who is disconnected from their illness, but emerge from the deep understanding that they are connected.

Human life has limitations. While it may not be due to cancer, death is inevitable. What is the sense in losing hope in life and worrying extensively about cancer? Rather, I believe life is far richer when a person gains consciousness of life's origin as a result of their diagnosis of cancer.

I feel that cancer survivors who truly comprehend the preciousness of their existence, who possess profound gratitude for life, and who are aware that illness itself is in fact 'Self' are the most fortunate.

III-5
The Voice of the Soul Reverberates in Cognitive Illnesses

Why does one suffer from dementia?
It is necessary to step back and view it from beyond the sphere of physical illness.
To seek what is vital to the soul.
Allow me to explain.

As the times change, all of life's concerns also change.

In former times, longevity was auspicious, something to celebrate, but these days, with each birthday celebration for our senior loved ones, there are hidden concerns. One of the biggest worries for families with members of advanced age is dementia.

Patients who are caretakers of their aging parents visit my clinic to consult about their mother or father being diagnosed with dementia. As someone with the same experience, I lend a sympathetic ear to their desperation with the quiet hopes that they will open up to the message that the illness of dementia is trying to convey to them.

I remember when my aging father, with whom I was living, began showing signs of dementia. There were small, apparently trivial signs.

For example, after I returned home from work, my father would sit me down to give me an explanation of his day down to the smallest detail. This was very much in character for my scrupulous father, who was a teacher during his active years. But listening patiently to these daily reports would invariably take a significant amount of my time. Once he was finished, I would let him know that I had taken note of all that had occurred, but as soon as I stood up to take care of my own matters, he would trail after me and begin a full recap of what he had just reported.

Had this occurred only once or twice, I could easily have dealt with it, but since he would repeat this daily without any sign of improvement, I would run out of patience, particularly after a long day at the clinic. I was concerned about my father, of course, and felt that I would have to adjust to his new behavior. At one point I put aside my preconceptions and allowed myself to simply experience my father's dementia-induced actions as they unfolded. As a result of immersing myself in that new reality, I was able to almost completely let go of the stress I had felt about his condition. As I now reflect on this time with my father, I am grateful for the helpful insight into the message of dementia.

When I am asked how one should interact with a family member with dementia, I don't go into too much detail about my first-hand experience. But I usually tell them this:

Although there will be many challenges, please open up your heart to them and let them know you are listening by saying, 'I understand you,' no matter what they say. They need to feel heard and understood.

How the person seeking advice on dealing with the dementia of a family member understands that last sentence depends on their outlook on healthcare and life, or rather their perception of life and death that governs their very attitude towards life.

Thus I don't feel certain that my words can be sufficiently understood. For example, those who only trust in Western medicine classify dementia as a type of illness, so they may believe it is sufficient to suppress the symptoms with medication or some other procedure. That is one way to view a human life, but that perspective will rebound at some other time in their lives when they are facing health challenges: if you treat another person as though they were a simple machine, then that is how you may be treated in a similar situation.

One has no choice but to either accept the possibility of one's own dementia, or convince oneself that you will never find yourself in that situation. This depends on one's lifeview, but since every one of us is part of the magnificent Mechanism of Life that spans a universe over 13.8 billion years, I suspect that if we view the illness that emerges at the end of one's life as holding a certain, necessary meaning, our lives will become richer.

So: why does a person suffer from dementia?

From the approach of Western medicine, the answer is that some kind of disability occurs in the brain, creating an anomaly in cognitive functioning. Brain disorders can be triggered by physical trauma such as accidents and strokes, or by atrophy of the brain itself. The approach of Western medical treatment of brain disorders is to remove the injury if possible, and stop the progression of atrophy.

As previously explained, this imputes a causal relationship limited to the solid and liquid fields of the body. When I speak of what a person with dementia needs, what emerges in the back of my mind is the vista you see when you step back and look at the situation from a distant place. That place is within each one of us and can be considered as the dwelling place of our souls that glows within the origin of our own Mechanism of Life since our birth.

As I mentioned, my father was a teacher in his active years, and as it is well known among care workers for the elderly, there is a subtle correlation between a patient's occupation and dementia. A survey of elderly patients with dementia reveals no shortage of participants who had worked in occupations in which observation of social rules were continually required, such as school teachers and civil service employees.

Of course, there are also many elderly who worked as educators or civil service employees who show no cognitive decline. And conversely, there were those with dementia who had worked in other occupations. The correlation between work and dementia is not complete. In consideration of those facts, I have a suspicion that my father actually wanted to do something other than be a teacher. Perhaps he may even have wanted to let loose and break free from the constraints of his job.

Regardless, since he was a teacher, he wouldn't have done so, and he must have had to suppress the voice of his spirit with reason for a significant part of his life.

Furthermore, I suspect some correlation with my father's suppression of his childhood feelings of craving his parents' love, so much so that he would do all he could to be the perfect child. As his son, I became a substitute for his parents, and it was my role to release him from the trauma he had experienced as a boy.

While it's only speculation, I imagine that those who take up careers that emphasize social rules give priority to what they feel they should be doing over what they would like to be doing. The will to take up a challenge or interest can be said to be the inborn voice of the soul, but often that voice comes into conflict with the voice of reason that is controlled by society. There are those who can still express their souls despite the clash with their socially driven voice of reason, but those who take up careers in which they must consistently obey societal rules may find it more difficult. Consequently, the voice of the soul dons the armor of the voice of reason and acquiesces, but once the binding of reasoning loses hold in one's senior years, the energy that had been censored up until then starts to overflow beyond the strictures of society.

There may be some Japanese healing practitioners who claim to treat illnesses of the soul, whether it be with traditional medicine or allopathic medicine. But it is certain that the concept of the soul has been passed down from ancient times, 'a source of life' that is uniquely referred to as a soul.

There is a phrase, 'the body is the cast-off shell of the soul,' which refers to the age-old idea that humans are not only composed of their physical bodies. We exist as human beings only once a soul inhabits the body. Owing to our souls, our feelings can be expressed with vivacity, and we can reveal our tenacious and beautifully brilliant spirits.

In that sense, the soul at the source of human life may be like the light of the sun. Just as all life on Earth thrives in the light that brightly shines down from the sun, the mind and emotions also thrive vigorously because of the power of the innate human soul.

To summarize my thoughts: if we can stand back and take a broader look from the vantage point of the soul, even with such an illness as dementia, we can see that an elderly person who has long suppressed the voice of their soul can finally speak with it. I keenly feel that dementia may be the voice of the soul.

III-6
The Formidable Power of the Subconsciousness

Why would they do this to me?
Why did they say such a thing?
When such questions suddenly arise, stop and think;
They may be messages from their subconsciousness.

The condition of a body that we call illness does not necessarily appear distinctly as a disorder of the solid and liquid fields of the body (i.e. the visible body); it can also emerge from the instability of mind or action, and only after reflection on the circumstances can one understand why.

You may have had the experience of a friend or acquaintance becoming suddenly ill, and it might have come to you as a surprise, since they hadn't appeared to be in any worse condition health-wise than anyone else. An unexpected illness reveals that some hidden problem must have been burdening them all along. In such cases, this type of illness may generally be considered an illness of the spirit or mind. But what is the primary cause of such an illness? A deeper investigation will usually lead to a field outside the invisible gaseous field of the body.

Somehow or other, the message of such an illness appears to come from the fields that control consciousness.

If this is the case, then it is vital that we first understand the properties of these so-called fields of consciousness.

As I mentioned briefly in Chapter 2, the parts of the body that control consciousness include two fields: individual consciousness (individual consciousness and subconsciousness) and hyper-consciousness.

The awareness that occurs within individual consciousness is also described in Japanese as 'manifest consciousness,' referring to the keenly aware state of existence. It is the primary consciousness that is the source of thought and self-will. This is what we generally mean when we use the term 'consciousness.'

The other field of consciousness is the subconsciousness. In Japanese, subconsciousness is referred to as 'latent consciousness.' This is the unaware state of existence, otherwise known as the 'unseen consciousness' or 'hidden consciousness.' When a state of illness derives from a problem in the fields of consciousness, in most cases, there is a causal relationship to a problem in the subconsciousness.

When a problem occurs in the subconsciousness, it affects the gaseous, solid, and liquid fields, and emotions and actions become unstable, influencing the physical body. While these are phenomenological correlations, the most troublesome aspect of subconsciousness is that its actions are taking place in an imperceptible field of consciousness that cannot be readily observed, even if one has the desire to observe them.

Since we generally perceive the world around us (as well as ourselves) by activating our manifest consciousness within the field of individual consciousness, this should be a place most familiar to us. On the other hand, we have no idea of the field of subconsciousness that spreads out around us. That is why we cannot easily detect a problem that has occurred there.

We can use a plant as our model for understanding consciousness and subsconsciousness. The part of the plant that is thick with deep green leaves is the consciousness, and the part below the earth, the roots, is our subconsciousness. If the roots did not serve an important role in sustaining the life of the plant, they would not be of much interest, but in fact it is the reverse. Without the roots to take in nourishment and water from the soil, there is no life.

Despite the extremely important role it plays in our survival, this invisible subconsciousness field is in fact similar to the roots of such a plant. If the word 'mind' can be applied as a collective term for the various invisible bodies including the emotions and the spirit, the subconsciousness can be considered the root of the mind.

Now, how do problems occurring in the field of subconsciousness manifest? The easiest problem to observe is when a single-pattern action is repeated over and over.

As an example, imagine that for some reason you feel dispirited after seeing the actions of someone we will refer to as 'Person A.' This particular situation does not have any correlation with your relationship with Person A, since you become despondent in the same way when the action is carried out by Person B or C. Even if it is not your intention to react in a certain way, your response is beyond your control. In such a case, it is likely that the cause lies in your subconsciousness. If you become low-spirited when you see a specific action by another person, you can infer a certain pattern within your subconsciousness.

Of course, you may argue that the reason you get dejected is because Person A is being overbearing, and that this is not necessarily a problem occurring only in the subconsciousness. Yet even if the person in question was overbearing, not everyone would react the same way—not everyone would be brought down by that person. There will be some people who aren't affected even if a person is bossy. When investigating the primary cause of a symptom that troubles you, it is helpful to consider that the pattern of a personal interaction is located within the subconsciousness.

Even so, there will be those who question this premise. They may question whether the subconsciousness can have such a strong influence on a person, or they may think that whatever they do, they are able to firmly act with intent. They believe that their reasoning is always fully engaged, and they cannot be swayed by the imperceptible subconsciousness.

Those who think that way may very well live out each day with firm intent, but the sphere in which the subconsciousness is active far exceeds the sphere in which we think in terms of common sense.

Now I would like you to recall your actions on an average day.

Perhaps your day will begin like this: you arise from your bed, open the window, wash your face, brush your teeth, and so on. While you are carrying out these motions, rather than being inattentive, you are aware of what you are doing. There is a tendency to believe that you are acting from your consciousness, but in fact, such behavior is entirely related to your subconsciousness. Your subconsciousness includes everything you have experienced in the past. Because your subconsciousness has made precise decisions based on those experiences, you are able to smoothly carry out these daily actions.

Your consciousness intervenes the moment an irregularity impacts your general routine. For example, you happened to invite a friend over early in the morning, and so instead of opening the window when you first get up, you wash your face instead, breaking up the usual rhythm of the day. This will probably leave you with a slightly odd feeling. On an average morning, there had been no need to give much thought to the motion of opening the window, but since your routine was altered, your consciousness took over and impressed upon your will the action of opening the window. If from this day onward you will have morning visitors, your subconsciousness will take over once again.

In this way, although you might imagine that you are behaving from a consciousness-driven decision-making process, in actuality your subconsciousness is active in the present moment, and actions carried out under its influence occupy a considerable part of your daily life.

Among the functions of consciousness, the subconsciousness or unintentional aspect of the mind represents around 90 percent of one's total brain function, and when thought about in the above context, this makes sense.[1]

In the example of a person who developed a pattern of becoming despondent in response to a certain behavior, initially this probably occurred independently of the subconsciousness. There could be any number of reasons such a pattern developed, but perhaps there is a correlation with the childhood relationship to one's parents. If the father was very authoritarian, he may have had a tendency to impose his way of thinking on the rest of the family, and thus his children would have been influenced by him to no small extent.

Once a child grows old enough to possess worldly awareness, they may get an urge to rebel in order to have their own say in how to live their lives. But if they are controlled too overwhelmingly by a parent, they may start believing their desires are futile and begin to lose hope. The moment those feelings emerge, the pattern of 'coercion equals dejection' or 'coercion equals anger' becomes imprinted on the subconsciousness. Unless one recognizes this pattern, it will continue repeating over and over like a broken record. Yet as one matures and the initial concrete experience that was imprinted on one's subconsciousness becomes a distant memory, only the pattern of 'coercion equals dejection' remains.

We are now left with the question of how one gets rid of a pattern that has embedded itself into the subconsciousness? Fairly recently, the deep trauma of people who have experienced tragedy during war or a violent accident has become recognized, and now general hospitals have departments for so-called psychosomatic illnesses. While it is encouraging that these psychological issues that once were socially stigmatized have gradually gained understanding, from my perspective as a healer, based on what I have discussed thus far, I must admit that many of the treatment measures are puzzling.

I imagine that most readers know someone who has been diagnosed with a psychosomatic illness, and it is likely that in most of those cases the treatment was to medicate. Those medications were designed to act upon the solid and liquid fields. I am aware that this medication is prescribed to control symptoms that can be detected in the body's solid and liquid fields. However, when there is repeated blockage to emotions and 'qi' energy, the cause of illnesses of the mind is not the solid and liquid fields (i.e. the physical body). Therefore, how can medicine designed to act on the solid and liquid fields treat illnesses that originate in the field of individual consciousness? The limits of medical treatment are evident in that they only serve to suppress the symptoms.

It is likely that the ancients possessed deeper wisdom in treating these types of problems of the subconsciousness than we do today. Looking back on history from a traditional medical perspective, there were various places in the world where methods to purify the mind (subconsciousness) were passed down as traditional remedies.

One of these methods is by word. Certain words are spoken to heal 'wounds' of the subconsciousness by discharging the vast information (idle thoughts and words) collected in the mind. One such method is Ho'oponopono, the ancient healing method of Hawaii, which has recently become well known in Japan. Its method is very easy—to purify the mind with four simple phrases. From a traditional medicine viewpoint, the invocation of certain words of *Shinto* prayers can also be perceived as a form of medical treatment.

Using the power of words to purify the field where the subconsciousness resides is a much healthier approach to treating psychosomatic illnesses than using medication. If one could purify one's field of consciousness through the invocation of words at any time, there would be no more need for medication.

With that in mind, what if we can yet further deepen our understanding of the subconsciousness?

There may be many approaches to this, but it is my belief that every path to this understanding will eventually converge in a singular principle, which is: to possess a feeling of 'gratitude' toward one's first experience of suffering.

Let's say that every time you try to start something new, for some reason your motivation fades away. But if you were to carefully focus on the sensation of the pattern that is troubling you, you may find that whenever you attempt to do something, the childhood memory of getting called 'good-for-nothing' returns. The face of your authoritarian father appears, making you freeze in terror. Those with such wounds embedded in their subconsciousness are the victims of acts of anger, making it natural for them to feel like failures. Yet it is possible to pause in that moment, to revisit that experience more deeply and to re-interpret it.

You may be able to realize that in those moments, your father entered your subconsciousness, creating patterns where any act of authoritarianism incites feelings of anger or depression. If you are then able to reinterpret that pattern embedded in your subconsciousness as a life lesson, you may become the sort of person who can be kind to other people.

You can also ask, for example, why your father imposed his own one-sided dogma without listening to your wishes. It can be very meaningful to perceive one's traumatic childhood memories from a different angle. For example, you can attempt to revive your childhood memories with an awareness of your father's own childhood experiences. In doing so, you may develop an outpouring of sympathy for your father. You may realize that when your father was a child, he was treated the same way by his own parents; the reason that your father enforced such strict rules for you concerning your education was because he never experienced what it was like to freely express his own feelings when he was young. Even once he became a parent it was impossible for him to display his affection by respecting the feelings of his own child.

Once you are able to understand that your father also had a pattern etched deeply in his subconsciousness, a different impression of your father will emerge that is different from the one of him as an authoritarian figure. And when you are able to arrive at a place where you feel sympathy for your father, it is there that you will find the words 'forgiveness' and 'gratitude' waiting for you like close friends.

On an average day we are unable to understand why people speak or act the way they do. When a family member or friend that we feel we know very well does or says something unexpected, we feel surprised and even betrayed.

Yet in such cases, instead of writing them off, if we imagine that something they are unaware of is acting on their subconsciousness, it is likely that we will find a clue as to why they acted that way or said what they did.

They may have some illness of consciousness that is trying to convey a message, but you are unable to find the hints in their words or actions. Are you ready to receive a message with sympathy? Is your own field of individual consciousness pure enough to receive a message? Those might be the sort of questions the illnesses of the individual consciousness field are asking you.

Note
1 Refer to the diagram 'The Relationship between Consciousness and Subconsciousness.' Here, the subconsciousness is interpreted as 90% of the brain capacity:80% of which is the subconsciousness itself and 10% , the base consciousness.

IV

Meeting the You that is to be Born

Carrying the Traditional Wisdom
that has Sustained the Beginning of Life

IV-1
What Causes Morning Sickness?

I have asked mothers who experienced severe morning sickness the question,
'During your pregnancy, did you have any conflicting feelings in accepting your child?'
Morning sickness and the mental and physical state of the pregnant mother are very closely related.

Children are born in hospitals.

I wonder how many people in contemporary society would think to question such a statement. At the very least, I guess that it would not be a majority. Yet it was not so long ago that childbirth in hospitals became common.

According to an article I read, for some time after the Pacific War ended approximately 70 years ago, very few Japanese women went to the hospital to give birth. In 1960, however, the number increased to approximately half of the population, and in 1970, it reached a majority. Of course there might be some uncertainty depending on how the data was collected to get those statistics, but generally this appears to confirm a change in delivery location from home to hospital.

This means that less than a century has passed since this change occurred. If we use the scale of the history of humankind, however, for tens of thousands of years, even hundreds of thousands of years our ancestors gave birth to children and reared them in different ways. And it is unquestionable that the way they lived led to our own existence.

These different childbirth methods occurred within the social context of a close-knit extended family. Both immediate and extended family members took part in this important occasion as a collective experience. When we look back on the history of lifestyles that has sustained human existence, passed down through the generations, we regain the fresh perspective that medical care is not the wisdom of medical experts, but rather is something we discover, cultivate, and harness throughout our daily lives.

As a matter of course, traditional medical care that had been cultivated through generations of experience was required at childbirth, and so those vital practices were forged into wisdom. Unfortunately, that wisdom is seldom implemented in today's hospitals. The purpose of this chapter is to share at least a few of those practices.

Although the moment of birth is something everyone has experienced, it is a hidden memory that cannot be recalled by those on the receiving end of the delivery. Even though the moment can only be clearly experienced by the person delivering the child, I would ask my readers to absorb the following chapter with the sense that you are going to meet yourself at the time of your own birth.

In doing so, I imagine you will be left with a feeling of gratitude for this circumstance that we all take for granted—that we are here, existing in this moment, because of our safe passage through that once-in-a-lifetime experience.

I will begin with a discussion of what is known as 'morning sickness.'

Morning sickness is often explained in Western medicine in terms of physical changes within the body, but of course such physical changes do not occur without reason. Whenever anything happens within the body, there is always a definite reason, In order to understand bodily changes, it is first important to know the basic cause for those changes. This is true when considering the beginning of life as well.

Morning sickness occurs because of the new life that dwells inside the womb of the mother. In other words, morning sickness is evidence that the child and mother are now connected. If you can hold onto this idea for a moment, it might change your impression of the 'distressing and painful' experience referred to as morning sickness.

Once, I had a visit from a female patient who had at one time experienced severe morning sickness. She told me that her child suffered from extreme depression, presenting her with endless daily challenges. She wanted to know what she should do. At that point, she had not yet mentioned anything about her experience of morning sickness during her pregnancy with that child.

But after learning more about her background I became concerned, and after her second or third visit I broached the subject by asking her if she had felt any resistance to being pregnant or to accepting that child in her life during her pregnancy

It's a difficult question to ask a mother face-to-face. But I persisted because I had already detected a hint of the underlying issue.

It may have partially been due to my unexpected directness that she seemed to have no recollection of any negative feelings about her pregnancy. But my question seemed to trigger something in her mother who happened to be with her that day. Her mother tried to jog her memory about that time. Eventually she disclosed that she had such debilitating nausea in her first trimester and that she was hospitalized for about six months; and furthermore, not long after the child was born, she and her husband got a divorce.

After hearing this, my suspicions were confirmed and I was able to make the connection between her nausea and her state of mind during her pregnancy. Later in this chapter I touch upon the fact that it is natural to feel a physical sense of incongruity during pregnancy, since physically speaking something foreign has entered the body and taken up residence there. That is one cause of morning sickness, but in fact the major cause is the mental and physical state of the mother during this period.

In this case, the patient stopped getting along with her husband at the onset of her nausea. She began to blame her discomfort on her child.

If she had been asked at the time if she felt any resistance to bearing a child, in all honesty she would have answered 'yes.' Perhaps the social pressure to have the child added to her apprehensiveness.

Ultimately, the child was born, and the mother's feelings of resistance to giving birth subsided, but the problem remained, now as a wound inflicted on the subconsciousness of the child.

If a mother is reluctant to give birth, her child senses it through their intimate connection from the moment it enters her womb. Since the rejection has already entered its subconsciousness, I believe that the sense that it is unworthy of life remains at the very core of its subconsciousness even after birth. When something stimulates that sense of unworthiness, symptoms of depression arise.

Those who practice traditional medicine or who live in a traditional culture often speak of the concept that the new soul of a child and the existing soul of the mother may conflict, and the conflict may generate a wave of disharmony between the two.

This may sound completely nonsensical to those who only believe in the facts created by conscious reason, but if we could raise our perspective to the stratum of the mind and its unseen layers, we can see that this way of thinking is more matter-of-fact than mystifying.

My patient's trepidation over giving birth, complicated by the failure of her relationship with her husband, eventually led to her severe nausea. One could say that because there was no exchange of words, the souls of the mother and child were in dissonance.

Nausea during pregnancy is very honest in its expression of the discordance between two lives. Even if there aren't any problems her relationship with her partner, a pregnant woman's anxiety about her pregnancy, whether because of its timing, because of the need to earn an income, or because she simply does not want to be pregnant, can result in intolerable bouts of morning sickness.

If we consider this phenomenon in terms of the human body-field, the child occupies its mother's womb in the first stratum—the physical body level. However, if resistance to this new life develops in the mental dimension of the third stratum, in conflict with the will of the Self, the discordance will be felt in the second stratum—the emotional level. Then anger is released, discomfort emerges, and we can see the 'nausea' of morning sickness as a physical message of anger. Just as accepting food into the stomach is a symbol of 'receiving,' nausea and ejection of food are symbols of 'rejection.' In other words, the rejection of the child is transferred into the nausea of morning sickness.

Whether it is as severe as with this particular patient, in this day and age morning sickness affects many women. In former times, when a woman became pregnant for the first time, it was natural to feel gratitude that one had been 'blessed with a child.' It would also have been natural for others to also celebrate the new life as a blessing. These days, however, many of my female patients ask me questions about their pregnancy, such as 'What should I do?', 'Am I doing the right thing?', or 'What food should I eat?' Hesitation is one factor that produces negative energy. When one is uneasy and resistant for no particular reason, light morning sickness appears.

If society were to become more encouraging and supportive of women raising their children, and if everyone eagerly embraced children, the child would be able to experience healthy human relationships from the time they were in the womb, and the number of mothers who experience agonizing morning sickness would significantly decrease.

The connection between mother and unborn child is integral. At the same time, a mother is connected to the father, to other family members, and to society at large. The issues that cause morning sickness are not only the mother's issues, but also the issues of those who surround the mother and the child within her womb.

As I posed at the beginning of this section, it is critical that we have a clear understanding of the phenomenon of nausea a mother experiences during pregnancy. It is not something that can be explained merely on physical terms, nor is it something to be loathed. Rather, it is a valuable message that the body is conveying—that one life has been connected to another.

IV-2
Where True Prenatal Care Begins

Gratitude for this day.
Gratitude for the food we eat.
Gratitude for the life that is born.
All of this is for the sake of prenatal care,
But there is something even more important.

The time when a child resides in the mother's womb as a new life is a special time for both mother and child. Until the child is delivered into the world, the mother and child have an intimate bond and live as one life, mutually influencing one another. This time demands careful attention; thus the emergence of prenatal care.

In Japanese, the word for 'prenatal care' consists of the characters 'fetus' and 'teach,' so some people think it has something to do with preschool education. Of course, this is not so. Instead, it refers to the wisdom that teaches a mother-to-be and her family what to do during pregnancy to support the well-being and healthy development of the life growing inside the womb.

Prenatal care involves the knowledge of a pregnant mother's ideal mindset, what to eat, how to care for and move the body, and all the other aspects of daily life during pregnancy. Every aspect of life is potentially part of prenatal care. For example, if the mother-to-be has a routine of giving praise for her existence every morning, and giving praise for the day every night, she is providing daily positive prenatal care.

Reading the Bible or books that encourage a positive and calm feeling also imbues the gestating child with positivity, and so is a wonderful activity.

If the pregnant mother eats high-quality, whole foods, her thoughtfulness will spread to her child as a positive message. On the other hand, a mother who, despite knowing better, indulges in food laden with additives cannot be considered to be providing good prenatal care.

The difficulty of prenatal care is that every aspect of a lifestyle can bear an influence on the mother and child—either positive or negative.

As I mentioned in the opening section of this chapter, the worst possible negative impact to an unborn child occurs when it receives the message that it is not welcome. In most cases, this occurs when the pregnancy was out of wedlock and unplanned. Perhaps if that situation leads the couple to marry, it will be different, but let's say they are reluctant to make the commitment. If the child is unwanted while in the womb, it may be exposed to arguments between the parents, and will suffer confusion at its mind level. If so, it may arrive into the world with a hidden misery.

As I said earlier, there is a tendency for children born under such duress to suffer depression, some quite seriously.

Such instances of trauma in the womb may be considered the worst-case scenario in prenatal care. It is heartbreaking to think of the challenges of a child born to parents who regret its birth. But in the soul-to-soul exchanges between mother and unborn child, it may also be that the child chooses to accept its mother and the circumstances it is born into. Perhaps in the child's previous life, it was the parent of an unwanted child, and it would like to resolve its past regrets. While of course it is up to my readers how to interpret these ideas, parents should certainly accept and welcome the blessing of new life, and firmly commit to that feeling until the child is delivered into the outside world. That is the most ideal form of prenatal care.

Generally, prenatal care implies a one-way focus of attention from mother to child, but if you shift your perspective a little, you can also perceive a flow of messages from a needy child to its mother. For instance, sometimes I hear expectant mothers say that their child is trying to tell them not to eat a certain food. One of my patients had a strong preference for vegetables, but once she became pregnant she could not suppress a desire for meat, and so she started eating it without really knowing why. But since she was not accustomed to the daily consumption of meat, she wound up suffering from indigestion. It was only after she became aware of this pattern that she realized that her desire for meat was a message from the child she was carrying in her womb.

In this situation, what is important is communication: the mother needs to acknowledge her own desires along with her child's, and let it know that on certain days she will be eating vegetables instead of meat. If she communicates clearly with her child, they will understand and be fine.

The sudden change in taste preference is also experienced by others, for example, organ transplant recipients. In the case of expectant mothers, however, the energy of the child's soul is making requests from within the mother's womb and so the influence is more extensive. It is not uncommon for an unborn child to also have an impact on the mother's hobbies and interests.

If there is a great variance in a woman's taste and interests after her pregnancy, such as: she used to enjoy walks, but suddenly stops enjoying them; or she formerly disliked pets, but suddenly wants one; or she had an interest in art, but now takes a stronger interest in music—perhaps this can be seen as the desire of the child growing in her womb. Doesn't that seem possible?

To those who are familiar with the principles of quantum mechanics, it is natural to think that the child's consciousness transmits information to the mother, whose consciousness changes in response, thus influencing her preferences and interests. However, I believe there are many to whom this may still sound magical. If you investigate thoroughly, you will find at the root the following phenomenon: the mother's energy and the energy of the unborn child, which are both particle-like and wave-like, interact with each other. If one side makes a strong request that goes against the harmony of the two energies, there will be movement in the direction of that request. As a result, it's quite natural that a mother's food preferences can change.

Through recent advancements in medical research, we know that the hormonal, immune, and autonomic nervous systems can be altered through one's consciousness, and that chemical substances play the role as mediators.

If a mother-to-be understands this principle during her pregnancy, it is likely that she can accommodate her child's food preference. If she wants to indulge her own food preference on a certain day, as long as she consciously communicates her intentions, the child will contentedly submit to her wishes.

With this perspective, one's concept of prenatal care will naturally change.

What to eat, how to live, and other good intentions of the first stratum (the physical body) are not what is essential in prenatal care. First and foremost, the mother should be aware that the soul of the child in her womb is constantly sending her messages, as should the father. In this way, we can hold regard for the child from the time of gestation as a human being, which is the ultimate approach to prenatal care; this is where true prenatal care begins.

If society as a whole comes to share such a viewpoint, our social environment will certainly improve drastically. While there are only a handful of obstetricians who hold these views about pregnancy, I anticipate that more will emerge from here onward.

IV-3
Breech Babies, Moxibustion, and Cesarean Section Deliveries

There are some who feel if all else fails, they'll just have a cesarean section,
and there are some who earnestly want to give birth naturally.
There are some who want to be healed by others,
and there are some who will make every effort to heal themselves.
That difference is strongly reflected in the results—
That is one lesson I learned from my healing experiences.

I often get patients who are expectant mothers approaching their due date. They want my second opinion since their obstetrician has recommended that they deliver their child by cesarean section (C-section), but they prefer to give birth naturally.

I imagine that most women would feel the same. Yet, I also understand why the obstetrician would recommend a C-section, and that is troublesome. My patients' apprehension and concern over not wanting a C-section are valid.

How should we think about the C-section, in which a scalpel is used to cut open the womb to assist with a patient's delivery? While those who prefer to give birth naturally will resist this method, lives may be lost if they refuse it.

The question would be different if there were no options, but since the C-section method is available when vaginal delivery is not possible for the patient, I recommend that she clearly understand the reasoning behind the doctor's decision and agree to the C-section.

On the other hand, I oppose the idea of selecting delivery by C-section for the sake of convenience—for example, merely because vaginal birth seems difficult. I would like for my readers to understand that, fundamentally, C-sections should not be necessary.

With this in mind, it is important not only for the expectant mother, but also for the couple together, to fully appreciate what pregnancy and birth entail, and try to imagine what the child in the womb feels when it is delivered by C-section. It is important for them to be mindful about the delivery itself, and if their intentions are firm, I believe that they can avoid the need to have a C-section. It goes without saying, it is my belief that episiotomies are also not necessary to aid difficult deliveries.

When I first began my current practice in Goi (Chiba Prefecture), an acquaintance who was an acupuncturist consulted me. His wife was pregnant, but she was found to have a large ovarian cyst. Although she had gone to various obstetricians for examination, the prognosis was that she should abort the child because delivery would be impossible. It was a very disheartening situation.

The ovarian cyst was found to be the size of a clenched fist. According to obstetrics, since they distort the form of the uterus, cysts impact the growth of the child. That is likely the reason for the harsh advice she was given. If the cyst is removed before the pregnancy, there is generally not any issue.

Once I fully understood the circumstances, I suggested a two-pronged approach. As she was a pharmacist, I told her to get a prescription for a good *kampo* medicine for the health of her and the fetus. Next, I instructed that she follow a diet centered on brown rice and vegetables (also known as a macrobiotic diet). Although fish, shellfish, and soy protein are good sources of nutrition, the basic daily meals should be macrobiotic. If the wife followed this proposal, then she would be fine. I assured her that I would also support her through her pregnancy.

As a result, a very healthy child was born without negative impact from the cyst. I feel that this is a result of the coexistence and resonance between the mother, the cyst, and the fetus.

I also have had consultations with expectant mothers whose obstetricians advised against natural childbirth because their first child was delivered by C-section, and it would be dangerous.

In the case where the firstborn child is delivered by C-section, it is safe to do the same with the second child—this is generally the accepted rule of thumb in Western obstetric practices around the world. The reasoning is that since the mother did not experience vaginal birth with the first child, the second birth would be even more complicated and rough.

Certainly that is one perspective, but there are many actual counterexamples that prove this is not always the case.

As long as the mother-to-be thoroughly understands the significance and reasoning behind the obstetrician's judgment, she should earnestly set out to improve the environment of her uterus, just as in the earlier example of the woman with the cyst. This requires good food, positive intent, and other lifestyle changes to create the optimal environment for natural childbirth. If there is enough serious effort, it will be possible for the second child to be delivered vaginally.

That being said, this is not an easy goal to fulfill, and if the mother-to-be is not determined enough, but only has a mild desire for a natural delivery, the desire is all she will have. If instead she makes a firm decision, her cells and uterus, indeed her whole body will cooperate in producing a suitable environment for a natural birth.

Obviously the process from pregnancy to delivery cannot be entirely determined beforehand. As I have illustrated, it is not true that if you have a cyst the fetus will not develop properly; likewise, it is not true that your second child must be delivered via C-section because your firstborn was delivered that way. While of course these should be considered as possibilities or risks, it is the nature of the body not to always respond in some prescribed way to a particular set of circumstances.

The will of the expectant mother and other family members, and the environment that she and her family create are critical to the outcome. What is also critical is the so-called education of pregnant women.

Prior to opening my current clinic 42 years ago, I had many questions about childbirth, such as why planned birth options and epidurals for painless childbirth were available, and so I extensively studied and practiced everything from kampo to moxibustion related to obstetrics.

In kampo medicine, there is a formula to support safe childbirth, and it is prescribed to pregnant women who are slightly anemic or where there is unease about the safety of the fetus.

In moxibustion, or the treatment by burning of moxa (dried Artemisia vulgaris, commonly known as mugwort) on acupuncture points, there is a method of treating a point on the leg called the San-inko ('Three Yin Channel Junction') from the fifth month onward to stabilize the condition of the womb and support an extremely healthy and smooth childbirth for both the mother and child.[1]

When my wife first became pregnant, I took advantage of the opportunity to practice what Dr. Ishino had taught me. (Although I would not presume to do so now, at the time I was quite bold in asking difficult things of her).

We centered meals in a macrobiotic diet, and from the fifth month onward we used womb-stabilizing moxibustion. I did not perform the moxibustion treatment, but I asked my wife to do it, as self-treatment enhances awareness of the life within.

After this child, we continued with two others in the same way, welcoming three healthy children into the world. Each time my wife worked right up to the day before her due date, so I feel validated in our efforts to test these methods.

There are also expectant mothers who are concerned about their babies becoming breech close to the date of delivery. These are cases where a cesarean delivery is performed as a last resort to ensure the safety of both mother and child. Before taking such a definitive approach however, I would recommend treating with moxibustion first, as introduced above.

There is a meridian point on the little toe of the foot called the Shi-in ('Reaching Yin'), and this is the meridian that works effectively on breech babies. For this point, I use a stick moxibustion that resembles a pestle.

Stick moxibustion is a type of moxa that is lit like an incense stick. To use it, you bring the lit end of the moxa stick close to the meridian without touching the skin directly. The treatment lasts at least 15 minutes for each leg, and the distance of the moxa stick should be adjusted during that time—drawing it back if it gets too hot, and bringing it closer again.

The duration of the treatment is key, because after applying heat for a certain period, the tissues of the womb will relax and loosen, and the breech position of the fetus will be restored to the cephalic presentation, or the head-down position. If the moxa treatment is too short, while the stimulus may improve the flow of *qi* to some extent, it will not be adequate to fix the breech presentation.

The posture of receiving the moxa treatment is also important; rather than a seated position, the method is more effective if the patient lies on their back with their knees lightly drawn up.

The effectiveness varies depending on the person, but for those whose bodies respond well to stick moxibustion, the breech will turn to normal positioning in a relatively short period.

There are several explanations for the breech position of the fetus; one is that the umbilical cord connecting the fetus to the mother becomes tangled, restraining the movement of the fetus. However, more often than not it is caused by the internal condition of the uterus.

Let us imagine that the uterus is the baby's temporary bedroom and the fetus resides there; since the room is filled with amniotic fluid, the heavy head of the fetus is naturally drawn downward and the legs become elevated. While this should be the most comfortable position for the baby, for some reason the state of the womb, its bedroom, becomes cramped or misshapen, forcing it to change position to become more comfortable, resulting in it becoming breech.

Among the reasons a baby may be uncomfortable in the womb is the misalignment of the mother's pelvis, or the presence of a tumor. However, if the problem causing the discomfort can be solved, the breech position can be corrected.

It may be easier to understand the circumstances if we imagine ourselves as a fetus.

Say that our bedroom is arranged neatly, so we can sit down in a natural posture without much effort. Now imagine that belongings are strewn around the room in a haphazard way and the room can only be entered by walking on your hands. If that is the only way that you can enter it, then you will remain in that upside down position until the environment is restored. That is the situation for the child in breech position.

There is another experience I had with moxibustion and a baby in breech position.

The aforementioned meridian, San-inko, which my wife used for self-treatment, is located slightly above the ankle on the inner side of the shin. This meridian is known to be deeply connected with the uterus and when stimulated properly will promote healthy uterus functioning. My mentor, Dr. Ishino, conducted research on recovering the fetus position from breech by cauterizing the San-inko with moxa.

When I first met Dr. Ishino, I followed his way of cauterizing only the San-inko with moxa, but soon after I became a licensed acupuncture and moxibustion therapist, I had a patient who consulted me on breech pregnancy. It was then that I began using the stick moxibustion to cauterize the Shi-in meridian located on the little toe.

That consultation came by way of a participant in a series of lectures I had been asked to give in Mitaka. His elder sister was pregnant and was due in a week, but had an acute kidney infection causing very bad edema. On top of that, her baby was breech. Her obstetrician had recommended a C-section, and she was to undergo surgery the very next day. Her brother earnestly pleaded with me to help correct the baby's position, so I gave him advice to treat the Shi-in meridian point on the little toe with stick moxibustion. I told him that if he alternated between left and right leg for at least 15 minutes each, after three days, the breech position should turn on its own. After I gave him the advice, I told him to notify the obstetrician; fortunately, when he did, the obstetrician delayed the plans for surgery by three days.

After the first treatment with stick moxa, the pregnant sister sensed that her baby had turned, but tests revealed that it had not. They continued the treatment and she felt a lot of movement on the second and third days. When they consulted the obstetrician to confirm, the baby had turned and the C-section was called off. On the following day, the fourth day of the treatment, I got a report that the sister had succeeded in having a very easy birth.

While the use of stick moxibustion on the Shi-in meridian was certainly effective, I feel that the expectant sister's tenacity and determination not to have a C-section was also a significant contributor to the successful result. Had she been nonchalant and passive about the treatment, without much ambition to rectify her breech situation, it is doubtful that she would have even followed through on my recommendation for using moxibustion. Moxibustion is most powerfully effective when the person using it has a firm intent; conversely, when used by highly dependent individuals, it is often not as effective.

The most important aspect of healing is not the patient's desire for healing to happen to them, but their passionate and earnest desire to do all they can to heal. When the patient's feelings of fervor and determination are transmitted to the body, they become great forces to bring about healing.

IV-4
Kampo Medicine for Babies
–The Effects of Digenea Simplex

Give Digenea simplex to a newborn to clean his body within.
A mother's first task should be to feed this to her baby
as soon as it is born.
If she does so, her breast milk is sure to taste more delicious.

A baby is born without incident—that instant of birth is a moment that overflows with relief and joy. This is an especially emotional time for those who have endured many hardships.

For the mother immersed in joy, her next worry may be about her breast milk. Will production be smooth? Will the baby nurse well? For any parent, child-rearing involves alternating moments of happiness and concern. But in regard to breast milk, I start with a discussion of kampo medicine for infants, which I hope will reach readers who are expecting or who are planning to have children.

This kampo medicine is called makuri in Japanese, or Digenea simplex. It is extracted from an algae known as red seabroom, and there was a time when it was mainly made from dried red algae from the seabed. Nowadays it is processed as an herbal medicine that is combined with rhubarb, Coptis japonica, licorice, safflower, and other herbs, and is boiled to be consumed as a decoction. In earlier times, it was known as 'kaininso,' and some may recall it as a medicine used to treat round-worm.

As you can probably deduce from its usage alone, it is a bitter-tasting medicine. Some feel the urge to spit it out right after they drink it. Its extreme bitterness is one of its characteristics, but also an aspect of its effectiveness (to eliminate harmful matter, as detoxification), and makuri is immediately effective when given to newborns. Infants who take it eliminate three times as much fetal waste as those who don't. Their meconium is black, consisting of all the fetal waste toxins that they absorbed while growing inside the mother's womb.

You may wonder why newborns have stools at all when they have not yet eaten anything. In fact, a fetus absorbs a variety of elements from the mother. Many of these elements are nutrients that are useful for development, but there are also harmful elements that are not used. These include byproducts of the mother's diet and emotional 'toxins' that cause trauma when absorbed inside the womb. Ordinarily, amniotic fluid is in a clean state without any harmful elements, but should the baby absorb amniotic fluid that was tainted by the mother's condition, the baby will also take in the harmful elements that were inside the amniotic fluid.

In other words, the infant must expel all of the harmful matter that they absorbed while in the uterus. For that, there is this powerful kampo medicine called makuri.

The Edo period physician Nanyo Hara (1753-1820) wrote in 'Sokei-tei iji shogen' ('Lectures on the Practice of Medicine' [A Mixed System of Old Chinese and Dutch]) (1803) that the name 'makuri' comes from the verb 'makuru' meaning 'to strip off,' with the idea that the meconium is gathered up and expelled. It was thought that infants who took makuri improved their suckling strength while nursing, had tougher skin, and would have more vitality, and thus it was given to practically every newborn during the Edo period (1603-1868).

What has happened to this miracle remedy that was so widely used in the Edo period? By asking experts around me, I found that very few obstetricians today know about makuri. And yet, this is an age where foods are packed with additives and people struggle with overwork and difficult relationships. The stress of modern life naturally affects the mother's body, as revealed in the pollutants found in samples of the amniotic fluid of pregnant women. The time to harness the power of makuri is even greater today than it was in the Edo period.

Perhaps it would be helpful to know how to use makuri. The recommended time to give Digenea simplex to an infant is immediately after delivery. Similar to the effect of fasting in adults, the body naturally cleanses itself of excess waste when it is empty, so the best time to administer the makuri is before the infant takes in a mouthful of its mother's milk.

It is also said that if administered right after the infant is born, it will be less resistant to the bitterness of makuri. Because the kampo formula for makuri contains Coptis japonica, which has a strong bitter taste, it makes sense that once the infant learns the mellow taste of its mother's milk, it may react adversely, causing it to spit it out. Give it to the baby before it learns any other taste; it should be the first action taken once out of the womb.

As long as the infant is fed the makuri decoction immediately after birth, you need only a small amount in a single dose. But in present-day Japan, hospital stays after childbirth can last up to one week, so I generally recommend a three-day administration of the makuri decoction. Even after a few days, harmful elements can enter the body of the infant through nursing, and so a single dose might not be sufficient to eliminate all of the accumulated toxins. Practically speaking, however, not too many infants will be receptive to this treatment.

Even in my case, we were not able to give two of my children makuri right after birth, and by the third day they were both refusing to drink it, spitting it out with aversion. Yet still, looking back on how favorably childhood went for them, I am pleased with the result.

In order to administer the makuri immediately after birth, one would need approval from their obstetrician. While many maternity homes in Japan would give their approval, not many obstetricians have heard of makuri as a kampo medicine for infants. There may be some hospital doctors who would give their approval once you reassure them that this medicine has been used safely for centuries, that there are no side effects, and so on. But there are also those doctors who are unfamiliar with kampo medicine and who are exclusively devoted to Western medicine.

At present, it may be frustrating to go along with the protocols of the obstetrician in charge. I recommend that expectant parents talk to their doctors about the possibility of using makuri, and if they show no interest or refuse to give their permission, look for a doctor who is supportive. That is a better use of your time than fretting until the delivery arrives.

Of course my own experiences with Digenea simplex have been favorable, but those around me have also had good results. This is most certainly one piece of kampo wisdom that should become more widely known and used.

IV-5
A Gift to Mother and Child

There is a recent increase in young mothers
who prefer to breast-feed.
In fact, suckling an infant supports its body into the next stage of
development.
Try to harness the natural form of the mother-child bond without
excessive effort—
This is my advice to new mothers.

Breast milk or infant formula? This is still an ongoing debate in Japan, but recently I have noted a shift in the consciousness of younger generations. There has been a dramatic increase in the number who wish to make breastfeeding an integral part of their childrearing practice.

This tendency to prefer breast milk over formula is also clearly reflected in the national survey taken by the Ministry of Health, Labor, and Welfare from data gathered every ten years. To illustrate, let's take a look at the numbers; there is a question in the survey asking what form of nutrition was given for the first three months after delivery.

There are three answers to choose from: 'Only breast milk,' 'A combination of breast milk and formula,' and 'Only formula.' In the most recent survey (2015), it was reported that 54.7 percent, or over half of the survey participants, responded 'Only breast milk.'

For the same question ten years earlier (2005), that answer was picked by only 38 percent of the participants. That is approximately the same percentage as the survey taken thirty years ago (1985), which was 39.6 percent. It is clear how significant today's increase is. The corresponding decrease in the percentage who responded 'Only formula,' from 28.5% (1985) to 10.2% (2015), further indicates the recent trend.

Through the latest research, it has become well known that aside from the nutritional benefits of breast milk, there are several other superior attributes such as the strengthening of the child's immune system and the promotion of the mother's postpartum recovery. However, this knowledge also results in an increase in mothers who try harder to breastfeed than necessary.

Although this tendency to do one's best is a strength of Japanese society, I think it is also necessary to consider its negative aspects. Imagine you have learned that raising your child on breast milk yields nothing but good results, and you look around and see that everyone else is thinking the same thing. If this knowledge only led to a healthy approach to breast-feeding, that would be fine. But if you become overly conscious about not producing enough milk, it could be destructive, even leading to mastitis. So my advice is to be cautious of trying too hard.

Since Japanese have a tendency to take everything too seriously, it should be mentioned that it is perfectly natural to have trouble with breast milk production. The most effective approach is to consult with a midwife or talk to other mothers about their experiences and make appropriate lifestyle adjustments as necessary.

With respect to food, for example, one key is to limit one's consumption of meat, dairy products, or refined sugars, since they can increase the incidence of mastitis. A well-balanced diet should be centered on grains, primarily mixed with vegetables and a modest amount of seafood and legumes. If these two dietary habits can be established prior to the baby's delivery, not only will breast milk flow well, but the mother will have good circulation throughout her entire body.

Another point is that as much as possible when nursing, the baby should be suckled directly at the breast for optimal production. This method of breast feeding relates to the mechanism of milk production; in order for the child to have ample flow when needed, they must send a signal to the mother. But that is not all it takes—simply taking the nipple in its mouth and sucking on it will not stimulate production.

The signal from the infant is transmitted by taking the mother's nipple into its mouth and 'biting down' on it using the jaw and tongue. To be more precise, it is not just the nipple, but the mammary gland that the infant latches onto while at the breast. There is a round hollow in the baby's upper palate that perfectly accommodates the shape of the nipple. Latching firmly onto the breast, the infant deftly 'bites down' to squeeze out the milk. Infants who nurse skillfully go through a process of trial and error to get just the right 'bite' to stimulate the flow of milk. This approach of recruiting the baby to cooperate in breastfeeding is also a good method to help with smooth production.

In fact, this manner of suckling the mother's breast to nurse is incidentally connected to the development of the child's chewing ability. The basic muscular motion of using the jaw and tongue to suckle is essentially the same for chewing food. In other words, through the act of suckling directly at the breast, the baby's masticatory strength becomes developed and naturally prepares them for the weaning.

This is why when breast-fed infants wean, they are able to chew 30 to 40 times as soon as they start eating. Drinking breast milk at the breast is more beneficial than drinking breast milk from a bottle, because masticatory strength does not develop properly with a bottle. Moreover, transferring the breast milk to a bottle allows the milk to oxidize in the air and reduces its quality. Although the nipples on baby bottles resemble actual nipples, drinking from them does not require 'biting' strength; the infant can imbibe by merely sucking on it, without much development of the chewing muscles. Needless to say, this means that once the infant starts to shift to baby food, they will need to learn how to chew.

Breast-feeding seems designed to prepare the child for its imminent growth. The more that we know about life and its workings, the more we appreciate the finer details of the Mechanism of Life.

Some mothers worry about when to start weaning, that is, when to end the child's breastfeeding phase. There are various approaches: some say you should try to wean after a year, and some say if the child still wants to nurse at ages two or three, you should extend the breastfeeding period until they display signs that they are ready to wean.

I have heard that the former approach is popular in the US and the latter is common in Germany. Weaning also means being able to separate the child from its mother, and some children are ready for this by the time they are one, while some children take about two years to fully wean. Due to the variation, it is my view that there should be no standard age for weaning; rather, we should cherish the unique qualities of each child. There is a chance a child will suffer from an injury (trauma) to the heart if they are forced to make a clean break from nursing merely to maintain some status quo.

A child will eventually arrive at the point where they are ready to stop nursing, and will wean themselves when you are least expecting it. Regardless of age, I feel it is best for the mother to patiently wait for the child to naturally become independent from the breast. This is what I recommend.

Finally, the mother's mindfulness when nursing is critical. If she is preoccupied with her smartphone or with unrelated thoughts while she is nursing, the child will keenly sense this neglect and may feel distrust towards her. The act of nursing is a time for skin-to-skin contact and for communication between mother and child. While breast-feeding, don't be misled by bad advice—the unified heart of the mother-child bond is what is important.

Note

1 These treatments are mentioned in a book by my acupuncture and moxibustion mentor, Dr. Nobuyasu Ishino, called *Josei no Issho to Kampo* ('Kampo Support for Womanhood') (Midori Shobo Co., Ltd.), on which I also collaborated.

V

Becoming Ill is Also Living

Towards a World without Healers

V-1
The Mechanism of Natural Healing Forces

If you catch a cold, just pop a few meds.
People who approach illness this way believe that illnesses are cured
by medicine.
They think that coughs and high temperatures are illnesses.
But is that truly so?
We received our instincts from the universe.
The time has come for us to truly use our consciousness.

When chatting with people about the world of illness and healing, I am often asked, 'Doctor, what is your ideal model for the medical world?' Without hesitation, the words flow straight out of my mouth: 'A world in which neither doctors nor healers are needed—that would be ideal.'

Each time I hear myself say those words, I feel I'm reaffirming them; they are not a transitory thought, but words that reflect my enduring and undeniable view.

In fact, only humans, among all living things in this natural world, require experts such as doctors and healers to take care of the mind and body. In the first chapter of this book, I discussed the simple story of my family dog that restored his health by fasting. All other animate beings on earth aside from humans—be it animals, plants, or microbes—have the techniques they need to take care of their own bodies.

Creatures that lack those capabilities have shorter life spans, and allow others to take their place. However, in the process of unraveling their force to create the circle of individual wholeness and its place in a network, cells that die gradually become absorbed into the surrounding soil, water, and air, and again become part of the circle of life. That is the cycle we are all part of.

Life and existence do not cease at the end of an individual life; while changing form, life is passed down endlessly, and is part of a grand circle of life.

Seen from the perspective of the entire universe, the same forces that create this circle of life also connect stars and planets to produce a single harmonized entity. For example, in our solar system, an assortment of planets mutually influence one another as they orbit around the sun to create an orderly wholeness.

I would like to call the power and mechanism that creates this universe the 'Mechanism of Life.'

And I would like to show how this 'Mechanism of Life' appears before us specifically, and to study how it manifests in the various cases that emerge in the world of medical care. These are the thoughts that have inspired the content of this book so far. Once again, in this final chapter I want to touch upon the power we know as the natural healing force.

I say 'the power we know as the natural healing force,' but while the words may be familiar, there is also the possibility they may be misunderstood.

For example, let's say there is a person who catches a cold and has a terrible cough and a slight fever. To get rid of the pesky symptoms, they go to the nearest clinic and fill a prescription for fever-reducing medicine and cough medicine. After taking the medicine, their fever goes down and the coughing subsides. This makes them feel successful in conquering their cold. And it seems that they are mistaking symptoms—such as coughing, runny nose, and fever—as the illness itself. If that's the case, then it's natural for them to think that once the symptoms are relieved, they've been cured. In any event, anyone can relate to the feeling of wanting to relieve the bothersome symptoms as quickly as possible, and thus the rush to get the prescription filled and return to life as usual.

However, for such a person, the natural healing force is not a force at all. In their view, what relieved their coughing and fever was the effect of the medicine prescribed by the doctor, and if they had left it up to the force of natural healing, then their symptoms would have only worsened. This view of natural healing is much more common than not. This is where the concept of the force of natural healing gets confusing; if natural healing is interpreted as 'to let the body heal on its own,' then misunderstandings will arise.

I referred to the superb curative skill my family dog had as a 'natural instinct,' and what I meant by that it was 'the naturally endowed, inherent ability of the dog' to heal himself. Similarly, the natural healing force implies 'the naturally endowed, inherent power within our bodies that impels us from illness to health.' If it is understood in that way, there will be less room for misunderstanding.

You could even say that the natural healing force is the great 'instinct' that enables our very existence, and can be considered the core intelligence of our bodies (or of our DNA). It is the inherent force that all of us have within our bodies.

That power is already in our bodies, and it is perpetually in motion, because the natural healing force originates in and is analogous to the basic power that enables the existence of the universe. In other words, similar to the cohesive unity of the universe, the holistic unit that is our body is brought together into a circle by that power, and in order for the networking forces that create the circles to function properly, it unceasingly makes adjustments.

One way that we refer to this force that unceasingly adjusts and maintains the balance within our bodies is the 'natural healing force.'

All matter and events of the universe are in perpetual motion, and as form changes with motion, the system of the entity sustained by natural healing force is also sure to unravel at some point. This is the state that we refer to as death. From a broader perspective, as I mentioned at the beginning of this section, life is not interrupted by the end of an individual system; death can also be seen as the beginning of a new system.

When you think about things in this way, you can appreciate that natural healing force does not act only when one is recovering from an illness, and that it is completely different from the force of allopathic medication that only treats the symptoms of an illness.

To begin with, it's an illusion to think that one recovers from illness by using medicine. Without the natural healing force working in one's body to keep it in good condition, not even a tiny cut could heal. Medicine does not heal the cut, but it may assist the natural healing force if, for example, it slows the flow of blood. (Of course, medicine is effective as long as it is used to produce a certain known effect).

The illusion that illnesses are cured by medicine is linked with the habit of confusing an illness with the symptoms that result from the natural healing process. Those who have read this book up to this point will already know that the symptoms of a cold, such as coughing and fever, are not the illness itself; rather, they are the phenomena that emerge because the body is recovering from a state of illness.

What role do symptoms play in healing? I would like my readers to give some additional thought to this.

For example, a cough is the violently expelling of the breath, and through that action, the body can discharge foreign particles (viruses, bacteria, dust, etc.) that have entered through the mouth and sputum that has accumulated in the bronchial tube. A dry cough stimulates the throat to produce moisture. A fever serves many roles, but one important one is to act as immune strength against viruses and bacteria. Fevers release sweat; although sweat is unpleasant and appears to have no purpose, it serves to eliminate internal toxins through the surface of the body. There is one more duty of sweat, which is to restore the fever-ridden body to its normal temperature.

If toxins accumulate in the stomach, how can you eliminate them? The body comes up with solutions: one is to eliminate them through loose bowels; another is to eliminate them through urine. Sluggishness throughout the entire body prevents the waste of energy with needless motion. The condition of the stomach and intestines declines, leading to a smaller intake of food, and energy that would have been used for digestion is saved (the strategy taken by my dog).

Cold symptoms such as coughing and fever are evidence that the natural healing force is acting to restore balance when the body cannot respond sufficiently to bacteria and viruses. The same can be said of other symptoms that occur with other kinds of illness.

Now that I have explained all of that, perhaps you know what it means to take fever reducers and cough medicine as soon as you come down with a cold. Since everyone has a body endowed with natural healing force, is there any rationale in taking medication to halt its action? The answer seems obvious.

The full expression of the natural healing force, this gift from the universe, favors our survival. The position of animals who know this force as instinct is in contrast to the confused position of us humans living in modern society who cannot control the medical technology that they created.

If there is a way to optimize human medicine and medical care, I think it is to support the body's natural healing force, which everyone is naturally endowed with, to the extent possible. I can't imagine any other option, and I am certain that all of you who are reading this book will also agree.

These thoughts about so-called medical science are, to me, the essence of traditional medicine. In the next section, I will present the concept of self-care that emerges from traditional medicine.

V-2
'Self-Care' as Another Form of Treatment

Yojo **is an ancient approach to preemptive self-care,**
With a 3,000-year history as one of the pillars of traditional medicine
in Japan,
Based on forms of nature and focusing on daily wellness as a support
for both mind and body.
Slowly and carefully take time out of the day
To apply the teachings of Yojo
In your regular routine.

In the previous section, I discussed the grand illusion of medication—how taking medicine to keep a symptom in check is not actually a healing approach. Yet it is human nature to want to hold onto this illusion. The term 'convalescence' refers to the period of healing after an illness, but there are people who, despite their thorough appreciation of its importance, will go back to intense exercising and eating regular meals to full capacity after only two or three days of bed rest. And since they haven't fully recovered, their body suffers from the unnecessary burden and their symptoms return. As expected, they will have momentary regret, but the next time illness strikes, the same cycle repeats.

In fact, the concept of preventative care is one of the most fundamental pillars of traditional Japanese medicine. It's the idea that instead of waiting for symptoms to appear before responding, a routine practice of wellness can prevent an illness before it establishes itself.

This concept is called yojo (lit. 'cultivation of life'), which translates loosely to 'preemptive self-care.'

The concept of yojo came from 'Yojokun' ('The Way of Culturing Life') (1713), a book by the samurai physician, Ekiken Kaibara (1630-1714), written in the Edo period (1603-1868) that is still very well known today. A sensation when it was published, 'Yojokun' was one of the most popular books of the era, so the concept of yojo is known to have spread widely throughout the nation. Its author, Kaibara, served the feudal Kuroda clan in Chikuzen (now Fukuoka Prefecture) as both a physician and a Confucian scholar. In addition to his own frail constitution from birth, his wife's poor constitution led him into deep research on materia medica (herbalism) and kampo (Sino-Japanese) traditional medicine. Based on his own life experience and practice, in his later years he compiled 'Yojokun' as a practical guide to preemptive self-care and health maintenance.

The origins of the concept of yojo, which were also part of Kaibara's studies, can be traced back to a source found in ancient China in a philosophy called yangsheng, which incidentally is written with the same Chinese characters as yojo, and thus carries the same meaning of preemptive self-care.

According to Professor Sha Shinhan, a proficient scholar of Chinese traditional medical philosophy and history, yangsheng culture had already begun before the birth of Christ in the Shang dynasty (c. 1600-c. 1046 BC). In the Warring States Period (c. 475-c. 221 BC), the concept of yangsheng was compiled into a manual of the Yin-Yang and Five Element Theories based on Daoism. An ancient Chinese medical text, Huangdi Neijing ('The Yellow Emperor's Classic of Internal Medicine') (c. 770-221 B. C.), contained the first collection of China's yangsheng philosophy. This means that with origins dating back to the Shang dynasty, the concept of yojo has a history of over 3,000 years, overlapping with the history of the traditional medicine of Japan.

It is thought that the yangsheng philosophy contained in the Huangdi Neijing was introduced to Japan around the sixth century. The first time the term 'yojo' was recorded was around 920 in a book by Sukehito Fukane (c. 898-c. 922) called 'Yojosho' ('Extracts on Cultivating Life'). This trend leads to Tamba no Yasuyori's Ishimpo ('Recipes at the Heart of Medicine') which we touched upon in the section on acupuncture. In Volume 27 of Ishimpo, the natural law of Chinese traditional medicine is described.[1]

The concept of yojo that gradually developed from the Heian period (794-1185) became popular in the Kamakura period (1185-1333) through a series of books on the subject that began with 'Kissa Yojoki' ('Notes on Drinking Green Tea for Self-Care') written by Japanese Buddhist monk Myoan Eisai (1141-1215), who is famous for bringing tea culture to Japan. Finally in the Edo period, Kaibara's popular 'Yojokun' was written.

In 'Yojo no Chie to Ki no Shiso,' Dr. Sha summarizes Kaibara's concept of yojo as follows:

In other words, yojo is useful not only as medical treatment for convalescence, but also for the prevention of illnesses. Even for people born with weak constitutions, yojo has an auxiliary effect that enhances their vitality. Yojo is indispensable to treating illness; yojo leads to longevity...

While this quotation shows why yojo became so valued in traditional Japanese medical care, its impact can be more concretely understood with the following metaphor.

Let's compare the intense symptoms of an illness to the weather. Imagine that it is like a typhoon in which the rainstorm gets stronger as it approaches. In order to protect yourself, you need to take preventative measures such as closing the storm shutters and bringing belongings inside that would otherwise get broken. In medical terms, let's say these are emergency procedures. In this way, you have taken the proper measures that you could, and, as a result, you were able to make it through the peak of the wind and rain. The following day, the blue sky returns.

If you are living inland, you may feel that the worst is over and you can go back to life as usual. But if you are living near the sea, you may have a different reaction. You may feel restless because the storm is still at sea, and you may feel the need to keep alert until the waves die down. You're concerned that the storm might be disastrous, since your house needs repair.

Even after the storm has passed, the waves are still high. If you think of the rough sea as your body after an illness, then perhaps you will understand the relationship between illness and your body.

Those who are impatient and take their ship out to sea when the waves are high are like those I mentioned at the opening of this section, who will go back to intense exercising and eating regular meals to full capacity while still convalescent. Even if the high waves are a nuisance, they can't be defeated one by one. A powerful energy field, such as a typhoon, produces a series of large waves which spread over the entire sea. (Illnesses are the same in that they spread throughout the entire body.) It would be lucky not to get carried off by the waves, but in reality, life doesn't work that way—that is frequently how the story goes.

Of course, this is just a metaphor, but when we carefully observe nature in this way, we can often relate the changes of state to those of our body, often without much effort. As we see in the history of the concept of yojo, traditional medicine is based on philosophies of Laozi and Zhuangzi and Daoism that respect nature. I believe the comparison of human forms and natural forms has also become the logic of the medical science of the East. This is a basic difference from Western medicine, which has a strong tendency to understand the human body in terms of mechanical causation. In any case, both the sea and the human body come from nature, and are thus virtually kin, so it is obvious that there would be similarities between them.[2]

The basis of kampo medicine is the harnessing of the natural healing force. One method is to eliminate harmful elements from the body so that beneficial elements can return. If that is the entire treatment, there can be some healing, but there will still be something lacking. In agricultural terms, it lacks 'soil preparation.'

When there is plenty of microbial activity in the earth, crops will be productive and the risk of being attacked by bacteria and viruses will diminish. The preparation of soil is, so to speak, the yojo, or preemptive care in agriculture. Because the soil in agriculture is like the body for human beings, the body should also be kept in optimal condition.

The place in the body where microbes flourish is the gut; keeping the bowels in good health is one of the keys to yojo. The gastrointestinal tract is not only affected by food, but is highly sensitive to thoughts and emotions. In other words, it is essential to maintain a lifestyle with good circulation of *qi*, like the passage of a comfortable breeze, in all aspects of life—food, clothing, shelter, and the mind and heart—in order to keep the bowels in a healthy state.[3]

I will not go into any detail about the actual methods of yojo, since starting with Yojokun, there have been several contemporary publications that introduce these methods. However, if I may mention one important point that can apply to any situation, it is to thoroughly appreciate every aspect of life. Valuing this practice each day would create a strong foundation for yojo self-care.

Life in modern times is always busy. Just as the Chinese character for 'busy' is comprised of components that combine to mean 'to lose one's mind,' if one lives out their days unaware of what they are doing or thinking or feeling, self-care can get swept up in the 'busy-ness,' and the soil that is our body gradually becomes weak and malnourished.

Some might respond, 'Well, that's why I drink smoothies and take supplements,' but each cell of the body works towards an harmonic association with the will of the entire body, which means that if you hastily consume the nutrients, your body won't grasp the meaning and thus won't make proper use of them. It is just as though you were busily working on an assembly line, mindlessly passing items from left to right, and in the end you don't even recall what part you were working on—similarly, your hasty efforts at nutrition will not lead to any meaningful results.

If you think of your cells as having lives and wills while they exist, it would be prudent to appreciate every mouthful of food, and to be cautious of your actions and words when you speak to others. Even if for a brief moment, take time out of each day to feel the signs of nature in the rays of the sun, a breeze, or the coldness of water. And on occasion, turn your awareness to your breath going in and out—the work of the body that has not once rested since we were born—and appreciate the state of the air gently moving in and out.

Even such small things give richness to daily life and are sure to improve mental and physical health. Yojo is also a form of treatment—

even on days when it seems easy to 'lose one's mind,' I hope you will remember this from time to time.

V-3
Who Should Heal Our Illnesses?

We bring our illnesses upon ourselves.
Once you realize this, your outlook on life will be transformed.
If all of us change our outlook on life,
society and the world will also change.
To be ill is also part of one's life.

'Medical treatment will take care of my illness. They're experts, so I should leave it up to them.'

They may not say it out loud, but every now and then I can read these words on the face of a patient who visits my clinic for consultation.

For example, a mother comes in to consult about her infant. She says that the infant often runs a fever, but medication prescribed at the hospital never brings it down. She asks me to do something about it—and so the medical treatment begins...

But a child who often runs a fever, but isn't being attacked by a bacteria or virus, has a problem more to do with their constitution and diet. I know that if I prescribe a medicine that will bring her child's fever down, the same condition will repeat itself until the mother makes adjustments to the child's lifestyle. (This is where yojo, or preemptive self-care, comes in.)

Thus, after finding out the child's food preferences, I convey the important points about serving meals such as not serving too much, and then give them treatment (sometimes via distance healing), after which their fever goes down the second, if not first time. But when this patient returns after three months or half a year later and starts to tell me that they are dealing with the same pattern all over again, I am resolved to tell them the following:

'I understand the desire to see an expert to resolve the problem. However, the real cause is your daily mindset and lifestyle, and you have control over your own child's illness. Patients who don't feel the need to heal their own children will repeat the same thing over and over. Unless you become more proactive in caring for your child, this is our last session.'

'We bring illness upon ourselves.'

Many will feel these words of mine are too harsh. However, as I mentioned in Chapter 3, those who feel the strong conviction that their illness is their own responsibility know that it is up to them to heal undergo complete transformations of lifestyle. Those who commit to living their lives fully despite their illness, and those who set out with determination will acquire a refreshing brightness and a unique strength. That is why I speak to my patients with determination and conviction. It certainly does not mean that I'm just pushing my patients away with the unsympathetic command, 'Go cure your own illnesses!'

Traditional Japanese medicine also postulates that if one brings illness upon oneself, one can also cure it by themselves. The roots of traditional medicine lie in the concept of yojo, which was introduced in the previous section of this chapter. The fundamental and essential approach of traditional Japanese medicine is to improve one's daily lifestyle through the methods of yojo self-care. I feel that the ideal form of traditional medical care, beyond the boundaries of east and west, is to share the responsibility of medical care such that traditional medicine supports the daily yojo self-care of patients while they incorporate time for illness in their lives.

Yet contemporary general medical care cannot exist without experts. In today's society, it has become status quo to entrust any and all afflictions to a doctor who is a specialist. In the case of Japanese people, cultural etiquette requires the utmost respect for experienced doctors, so it might seem rude to attempt one's own healing rather than to leave the cure completely up to the doctor.

It would be one thing if upholding cultural codes of conduct led to favorable results, but since today's medical community has been co-opted by the profit motive, we have unwittingly placed our lives on the line in the name of big business. No doubt you have heard about pharmaceuticals and vaccinations that stealthily slip through legal loopholes despite widespread public concern about their dangerous side effects. If only the public organizations that should be protecting the lives of their citizens would make transparent decisions, we would not be forced into playing hide-and-seek with the hidden truths of our healthcare system.

After all, even if medical care is intertwined with corporations, ultimately we are responsible for protecting our own lives. Once we firmly acknowledge this, we should be able to make our own decisions about using medications or vaccinations.

Lacking the ability to make these decisions and entrusting our lives to experts is tantamount to being robbed of our own lives. First and foremost, I feel that medical specialists and professionals and medical patients should share in the decision-making processes to determine an ideal model for health care.

These issues of trust in allopathic care may naturally lead some to choose acupuncture or kampo medicine instead—a choice I would love to be able to endorse without ambivalence, but sadly, the situation with traditional medical experts has its own share of challenges. Even among those who run *hari-kyu* (acupuncture and moxibustion) or kampo medicine practices there is a majority who approach treatment symptomatically, just like they do at general hospitals. Far from serving as support, there are even healers who go around self-promoting that they have cured this or that illness.

I am able to recommend kampo medicine because there are few side effects, but regardless of whether you visit a general hospital or an alternative clinic, you must have a firm conviction that your illness is your own responsibility, and you are the one to cure it. The advice and opinions of the specialists are to be valued as nothing more than information for you to use in making your own decision.

What all this boils down to is that illness is both a personal issue and a social issue. If the medical system of a society is in a sickly state, it will affect individuals who are influenced to put their lives into the hands of others, to their detriment. Conversely, if the individual has an unhealthy lifestyle which results in chronic illness, so will society. A consumerist society has a negative effect on the global environment, and of course this impact extends to the rest of the universe as well.

Once you perceive the world as being full of like forms, you can understand a number of things in sequence. When you use a macro perspective to look at the world, your understanding will grow to encompass your individual self, your family, your community, your nation, your Earth, and finally, your universe. Conversely, if you use a micro perspective, you can reduce yourself to your cells and genes, and once you arrive at the smallest elementary particle, you can see that all of these entities share similar forms both as a continuation and a way of existence as life.

Every kind of life in this world exists simultaneously as an independent unit and as a part that fulfills a role within a whole. The collection of parts may make, for example, a nail on a fingertip, an eye, or a nose. But when the aggregation of collections of parts becomes a whole human body, the life of each individual part becomes part of a life on another dimension. A unique dynamic is born there doesn't exist anywhere else.

This nothing-less-than exquisite power of the cooperative—this wondrous world of networks—is truly amazing.

In other words, the foundations of the lives of each of us are in resonance with the vast undulations of the life of the universe. When we are able to appreciate that resonance, and allow ourselves to be moved by it, and accept illness also as part of one's life, our perspective of illnesses may be greatly transformed.

V-4
'The Four Inevitables' (Birth, Aging, Sickness, and Death) and *Shiseikan*

When you reach the intuitive awareness of your imminent death will you have an 'invisible walking stick' to lean on?
Do you have an idea of how to spend your final days?
Dying is not only about grief and sorrow.
Wouldn't it be ideal to say this with certainty?

Death is certain.

Although we may be able to comprehend this in our minds, will we be able to accept our fate without hesitation in the moments before the final curtain falls? Will I? Will anyone else? We cannot know the true answer until we arrive at that point.

But when the time approaches, will we have an 'invisible walking stick' within our hearts to carry us through? If so, our way of life will begin to change when death is imminent. In my many years working as a physician healer, I have shared the final days of many patients, and these are my impressions.

What will you use for your 'invisible walking stick'? Some will think of their family. Some will turn to a deeply trusted faith. Each person must choose their own 'stick.' But if every 'stick' has one thing in common, it can be summarized as shiseikan, or one's perception of life and death.

What does it mean to live and what does it mean to die? In Japanese, shiseikan is the concise word used to describe the thorough investigation of these questions. Because so much is encompassed in this investigation, the term is necessarily short.

Buddha, who said that 'Everything in life is suffering,' referred to shorobyoshi (birth, aging, sickness, death) as shiku (the four sufferings). Just as the term shiku-hakku (four sufferings, eight sufferings) is still used in Japan, Buddha's shiseikan of suffering has a universal appeal even today. However, I don't think that that is all there is to shiseikan. Rather than viewing the 'four inevitables' as forms of suffering, on the contrary, I believe there is a shiseikan that experiences the 'four inevitables' with gratitude and replaces suffering with joy instead.

If you have read this far, you must have developed a firm response to its main theme of illness, one of the 'four inevitables.' Far from a suffering that you should get rid of immediately, the pain and suffering caused by illnesses are a sign that the natural healing force is working to return your body to health. Once you accept this concept, feelings of gratitude for your hard-working body, as well as for the natural force (the Mechanism of Life) that gives your body strength, will well up inside you.

Granted, not all illnesses are equal. There are some illnesses that you can prevent with yojo, and there are some illnesses in which the body is disabled by a birth defect or an accident. When social problems such as starvation or war befall an individual, these may cause an illness. Not everyone is born under the same circumstances, and this brings unresolved feelings. How can we accept such illnesses as part of life? This is the big question. There may be more than one answer to this, but one thing can be said for certain, which is: if one could affirmatively accept their birth into such an environment, and all of their life experiences (otherwise known as 'fate'), at that very moment feelings of pain will surely be replaced with gratitude.

Similar words have been used in each of the mythical stories of ancient religions of Japan. For example, in the worldview characterized by a belief in transmigration, there are stories about how the past life of a person's soul can influence the present life. The Buddhist idea of karma (in Japanese 'go') also presents similar stories, but karma can also be regarded as a law of spiritual cause and effect. The account of karma is that the soul, independent of a physical body, determines how its next life will be experienced in succession to a past experience. For example, if someone is born with a disability or is born to abusive parents, there is some reason why that person's soul chose these circumstances. This leads to the idea that one's purpose is to become fully aware of the reason he or she was born.

Whether or not you subscribe to such a view of life, it is certain that the very instant you become aware of the reason such an illness was brought upon you—be it a karmically inherited one, a wound you acquired after birth (including any kind of trauma), or some relatively light illness acquired by your lifestyle habits—all of your feelings will be replaced with gratitude and you will appreciate your illness with a sense of joy.

As for me, I am fond of the idea that my soul chose to be born as my present self. As I have mentioned previously, life itself cannot fundamentally be divided into life and death. If the life to come is contained within one's present life, it is very natural to imagine that the beginnings of our present life had already existed in our past lives.

One's present fate (one's life) was chosen by one's soul. The wonderful thing about that concept is that once it is accepted, one will become driven with the determination and resolve to overcome one's challenges.

Suppose, for example, that you have extremely negative thoughts about your parents, that they deny you everything you want and only cause you trauma. At that point, you wonder why you were born to such parents. Taking another step deeper into the question, you say to yourself that this is the path you chose, that you were the one who decided to be the child of such parents. And once you can hold this thought deep in your heart, no matter how many times you want to escape from all the pain, once you truly leave home and start a life independent from them, you will be deeply stirred by all that you have experienced—and I think that moment is the moment when all previous suffering and pain turn into delight.

The suffering of aging: that concern may be one of the most representative of the present age. However, to see aging as misery is just one way of looking at it. The body doesn't move with as much agility as it did in one's youth, but conversely, by taking the time to think slowly and carefully without moving, one is able to look back on all of one's many experiences and reinterpret their significance. A time of calm introspection can only be enjoyed in one's advanced years.

As a result, the elderly can deliver the lessons that one has learned and the thoughts that one wants to pass on to the next generation. This is the role of aging. And it is an extremely vital role for society that can only be done when one is old.

Our lives do not consist of things that are wonderful and things that are meaningless—in fact, everything in life has meaning. This is our gift from the universe, and it is also the fullest understanding of the meaning of the Mechanism of Life.

The suffering of death: this refers not to the pain of death itself, but to the pain that comes from the fear of death.

As mentioned above, if we understand the Mechanism of Life from which the universe is constituted, life and death are connected and each is a continuation of the other. Even if we exist as a physical body for only a limited time, our bodies return to the earth, and our souls pass on to the next life.

While it is human nature to brood over one's own death, when the final moment approaches—whether it be for someone with an incurable disease, or someone without—there will be some kind of sign. At the moment of knowing, the soul will quickly review our life and reveal it to us. People who have had near-death experiences have spoken of revisiting their past memories like a series of flashbacks, and this instantaneous vision may very well be a signal from the soul.

If there is no time to revisit one's memories before the soul leaves the physical body, all of the emotional memories transfer to the ethereal body. This is how the soul allows the family and friends to sense these emotional recollections, as the soul announces its departure to a new life and transmits its gratitude.

Have you not heard stories of those who went before us who notified those around them when they realized their 'next destination,' and told them of their wonderful final moments in visible form before they went on their journey?

There is a well-known story of the death of the world-famous Indian yogi, Paramahansa Yogananda (1893-1952). Yogananda selected the day of his own death (March 7, 1952). Far from being sick, he attended a dinner that was held in his honor that day. After delivering a speech at his seat, having determined that he had fulfilled his role in this world, he entered a meditative state and consciously exited his own body.

It is not only Yogananda who is able to realize his own death and make preparations toward the appointed time; to varying degrees, this is something that anyone can do. Let's say that the final day is approaching, but there is a certain someone that the dying person is eager to see. They had been given only one more week to live, but once they set their mind to it, they are able to extend their lives by one more week. However mysterious this may sound, it is a fact.

What should you do when you sense your departure time is nearing? What is the most ideal way to spend those last days? This is my suggestion: The first thing is to reduce food intake. If possible, you should refrain from consuming any food and only drink water, a so-called water fast.

That way, the mind and body together enter a state of calmness. Even for those with some dementia, the symptoms gradually disappear. And, this I can say from experience, the person who reaches such a mental and physical state begins, without fail, to put their affairs in order two or three days before their death. Those who like books started to arrange their books. Those who taught traditional Japanese tea ceremony or flower arranging, they began to organize their kimono.

Presently, the time arrives. On the day of or the day before death, invite family and friends to spend the last moments together in happy reunion. Offer words of thanks to each person who helped you through life, and exchange your parting words. The time where both acknowledge that the end has arrived becomes the final farewell.

I refer to these last days together as 'the parting ceremony.' This time of parting, when we see off the person who is meeting their death, is not just the last moment of parting; in a sense, it has already begun for everyone, now, in this present moment; but it is in the days of 'the parting ceremony' when it is expressed in clearly visible form.

For those who share their final days with close friends—who go through the process of putting their affairs in order, exchanging final words of gratitude and farewell, and heading into the final journey—their departure is full of peace.

Of course there are those who meet a sudden death and are thus unable to even talk with loved ones at the end of their lives. In these cases, there are strong feelings of regret felt by the family left behind. Naturally, the way that death is accepted by those who have departed and those who have to continue life without them is different. However, it is said that even in the case where it appears that death was sudden, the soul of that person senses that the final days have arrived. I also sympathize with this.

Life is connected to death, and life is connected to life, in uninter-rupted continuity—perhaps recalling this idea each day will create a force that will gradually dissolve our regrets.

If the fact that we exist here and now is to be understood as a gift from the Mechanism of Life from which the universe is constituted, the four inevitable sufferings are the meeting places where irreplaceable encounters teach us that fact. At the place where this truth is felt, I imagine there will be an entrance opening onto the path to a new outlook on life and death.

I want to live out my life in gratitude for each moment and in awe of the splendor of the Mechanism of Life that allows me to exist. How about you?

Note

1 In Dr. Sha Shinhan's 'Yojo no Chie to Ki no Shiso' ('Health Care and the Concept of Ki') (Kodansha Ltd.), the fascinating interrelationship of Chinese and Japanese traditional medicine is described in great detail. (For those who are interested in the history of medicine in Japan, I recommend this book.)

2 Dr. Masakazu Tada (1911-1998), who thoroughly researched such subjects as the contradictions of Western medicine, the philosophy of Laozi and Zhuangzi, world religion, and philosophy, advocated traditional medical care and wrote extensively about the importance of preemptive medical care based on 'immediate health care' and the way of yojo.

3 In 1947, Japanese biologist Dr. Kikuo Chishima (1899-1978) presented a novel theory that blood is produced in the small intestine, which attracted attention in the 1960s. This theory challenged the conventional theory that blood cells are formed in the bone marrow. Along with finding great interest in this theory, my own experiences have led me to believe there is a need to study the 'intestinal hematopoiesis theory,' but it has yet to be formally accepted as a scientific theory. Disappointing as this may be, of late, despite all of the advancements made in scientific research on the gut, it has been found that there are still a vast number of unexplained factors in intestinal functioning. Japanese scientist and author Dr. Keiichi Morishita also supports the theory that blood is made in the small intestine, and I expect more progress to be made in this field of research.

Afterword to The Mechanism of Life ('Great Preciousness of the Source')

Everything began with a desire to write a book on the essence of medicine. With the intention for a book that would unlock a new outlook on medical care and prove useful for those receiving medical treatment, I searched for a phrase to best express its central theme. After about a year of deliberations with the editing team, appearing in the outer layer of my consciousness as if in a dream were the title words of this book: 'The Mechanism of Life.'

When I shared this with Dr. Kenji Nanasawa, he presented me with a special name. The name is 源大貴 (lit. 'Great Preciousness of the Source'), and it is written using majestic and beautiful calligraphy writting.

It was Dr. Nanasawa who suggested to me a perspective of the human body, an outlook through each of the five strata of the body's elements—body level, emotional level, mind level, interactive level and divine will level which I touched upon in the main text. This perspective washed away uncertainty and gave order to my ideas.

I learned that the concept of five strata of the human body exists in the *Shirakawa Hakke Shinto*, a sect of the native Japanese Shinto religion, of which Dr. Nanasawa has been a long-standing scholar.

Although I am not in a position to explain about the concept, my humble understanding is that the tenets of Shirakawa Hakke Shinto are not what we would today refer to as religious. Instead, I believe they were a systemized code of conduct, used for the ancient imperial family to reign peacefully without wasted efforts. These codes came from information compiled from the highest sources of knowledge available and were woven into stories and condensed into oral and visual form.

I apologize to my readers for my superficial understanding of such depths. Dr. Nanasawa, however, is an expert who occasionally conducts ancient rites, one of which is a special naming ritual for things and people. While not concerned with the timing and style of these rites, in keeping with the Japanese saying, 'Intuition is divine will,' Dr. Nanasawa presented me with the magnificent name, likely conceived on a whim.

While admiring the flow of the brush writing of the beautiful name I was presented, something immediately came to mind—that these were the characters to be given to the Mechanism of Life. Dr. Nanasawa, being an unaffected person, selected characters that held multiple connotations not seen on the surface. As a healing practitioner, I first take time to feel new ideas, including characters, with my body before trying to understand them intellectually. For example, when teaching students how to use acupuncture needles, I always tell them that before treatment they must first grasp what the life of the patient is demanding and in which field or stratum its origin is located. Then, they must sense how the needle wants to be used. Once one can separate from Self, they can use the tools of acupuncture free from bias.

This was a similar moment when I saw the new name that Dr. Nanasawa had suddenly handed to me. When trying to determine what these elegantly written characters were telling me, I was struck with an understanding.

When broken down into characters, this name can be interpreted as 'the Great Preciousness in the Source (of Medicine).' With that reading in mind, I decided to give it the same phonetics as いのちの仕組み (inochi-no-shikumi), or the 'Mechanism of Life' in Japanese.

Dr. Nanasawa had also explained, 'If you take the 己 from your first name and insert it between 大貴 , then you will get the name 大己貴 Onamuchi, the name of a deity.' As I mentioned in Chapter 2, Onamuchi is known as the deity of magic and medicine, and so it is a name that carries a lot of significance. Using the characters from my first name, one more reading that I arbitrarily added is, 'To revere (貴ぶ) the Mechanism of Life of the Grand Self (大いなる己) beyond Self (克己) .'

I recognize such a name for myself and my clinic is more than I deserve, and instead choose to interpret such an honor as Dr. Nanasawa's strong encouragement that I devote myself to the path of trials and tribulations of my work. It was thanks to these receiving these auspicious words from Dr. Nanasawa on the occasion of the publication of this book that I was able to climb this great mountain.

Personal musings aside, I would like to say that Japanese traditional medicine incorporates the science of life that is nurtured from all aspects of our daily lives. It extends to the customs and life wisdom fostered through the dealings and culture of what today is considered religious teachings and events. The significance of connecting to wisdom cultivated in ancient times will certainly increase as time continues.

Western medicine is but one outlook on medical science; in this Grand Ultimate world, it is time to revisit the concepts conveyed throughout this book.

It is time to aim towards integrative medicine.

And now, before I run out of space, I must thank everyone who lent their support and help towards the creation of this book.

I am incredibly indebted to Dr. Nanasawa, for whom I set aside overused words of gratitude for the diligence with which I will apply to my work going forward.

As I described in the foreword, the editorial staff of Waki Publishing Corporation supported me patiently for over two years, helping me bring this material together in book form. My deep gratitude to Hatsuka Funahashi, Hiroko Matsubayashi, Kayo Kato, the now independent Kiwako Araya, and finally, the president of Waki Publishing Corporation, Taisei Sato. I hope that you will continue to offer books to a great number of readers on the ideal path for medical science and medical care.

This book is a distillation of what I have learned from the many people I have been involved with as a healing practitioner, but for lack of space, I thank Dr. Toshiharu Koike of the Toumeido Acupuncture Clinic.

Dr. Koike assisted me faithfully during production meetings for this book, never complaining despite these considerable efforts. So that the production team wouldn't wreck the ship by the self-serving remarks of the captain, at times he would launch a lifeboat, or would lead the ship to tighten a hold on the course. Those on the editorial board of Waki-shuppan are well aware of his great contribution. Because it is up to his generation to create a new traditional medical care, I anticipate much more activity in the future.

Finally, I would like to offer gratitude to my beloved family.

From the time I opened my clinic in our hometown of Goi, I have been able to lead a busy life as a healer giving lectures and instruction all around the country thanks to the constant support of my family. Many years have involved forgoing annual family vacations to prioritize treatment of those in need. While my words of gratitude are coupled with words of innumerable regrets, this is the life of a healer. If I can put down the words 'thank you,' which I normally have trouble saying, perhaps that will earn me their pardon for a while.

I now close this book with the hopes that the blessings of the Mechanism of Life will visit everyone who takes this book in their hands.

On an auspicious day in March 2019
石原克己
Katsumi Ishihara

Kazumi Ishihara, Healing Practitioner

Born in 1950, Chiba Prefecture, Japan

After graduating with a degree in Pharmaceutical Sciences at Tokyo University of Science, Ishihara Ishihara completed studies in *hari-kyu* (acupuncture and moxibustion). Extending beyond the field of medical science, as a highly skilled and distinguished acupuncturist and healing practitioner, Ishihara widely pursues the essence of the Mechanism of Life through his clinical work, mentorship of other practitioners, as a lecturer, and a public speaker. Ishihara is particularly noted as a successor of kyu-shin (or 'nine-needle' acupuncture), an ancient acupuncture method, which has become nearly obsolete in its origin of China.

Bibliography

In this bibliography, I list works referred to in this book in the 'References' pages and works suggested in 'Further Readings' pages.

The works' detail is provided in the following order: the author's name in Japanese, its pronunciation, published year, book title, its pronunciation, meaning in English and publisher. Note that this is a basic format. The works on the lists do not necessarily follow this order or are provided with all information.

References

Chapter I
Fulford, Robert. C. (2001). *Touch of Life: The Healing Power of the Natural Life Force*. Gallery Books.

Chapter II
大同類聚方 *Daido Ruiju Ho.* (808).
杜思敬 Du, Si. Jing. (1965). 鍼經摘英集, *Zhen Jing Zhai Ying Ji.*
淮南子*Enanji*. (n.d.).
福岡伸一 Fukuoka Shinichi. (2009). 動的平衡　生命はなぜそこに宿るのか *Doteki Heiko: Seimei waa Naze Soko ni Yadoru noka* [Dynamic Equilibrium]. Kirakusha.
Gerber, Richard. (2001). *Vibrational Medicine*. Bear & Co.
古語拾遺 *Kogo Shui* [Collection of Ancient Stories].(807).
古事記 *Kojiki* [An Account of Ancient Matters]. (712).
老子 *Laozi*. (n.d.).
列士 *Liezi*. (n.d.).
日本書紀 *Nohon Shoki* [The Chronicles of Japan]. (720).
丹波康頼 Tamba no Yasuyori. (984). 医心方, *Ishimpo* [Recipes at the Heart of Medicine].
角田忠信 Tsunoda Tadanobu. (2016). 日本人の脳 理性・感性・情動、時間と大地の科学 *Nihonjin no No: Risei, Kansei, Jikan to Daichi no Kagaku* [The Brain of the Japanese: Reason, Sensitivity and Emotion, Science of Time and Earth]. Taishukan Publishing Co., Ltd.

東京九鍼研究会 Tokyo Kyu-shin Kenkyukai. (2012). ビジュアルでわかる九鍼実技解説 *Visual de Wakaru Kyushin Jitsugi Kaisetsu* [Nine Needles Techniques in Visual]. Midori Shobo. Co., Ltd.

Chapter IV
石野信安 Ishino Nobuyasu. (1984). 女性の一生と漢方 *Josei no Issho to Kampo* [Kampo Support for Womanhood]. Midori Shobo Co., Ltd.

原南陽 Hara Nanyo. (1819-1820). 叢桂亭医事小言 *Sokeitei Iji Shogen* [Lectures on the Practice of Medicine]. Shitamachi Honcho (Mito), Suharaya Yasujiro.

厚生労働省 Ministry of Health, Labor and Welfare. (2015). 平成27年度乳幼児栄養調査結果の概要 *Heisei 27nendo Nyuyoji Eiyo Chosa Kekka no Gaiyo* [The Summary of Infant Nutrition Survey Results in 2015]. Employment Environment and Equal Employment Bureau and Child and Family Policy Bureau, Ministry of Health, Labor and Welfare.

Chapter V
貝原益軒 Kaibara Ekiken. (1713). 養生訓 *Yojokun* [The Way of Culturing Life].

黄帝内經 *Kotei Daikei*. [The Yellow Emperor's Classic of Internal Medicine] (B.C.770-221).

深根輔仁 Fukae Sukehito. (n.d.). 養生抄 *Yojosho* [Extracts on Cultivating Life].

謝心範 Sha, Shina. (2018). 養生の智慧と気の思想 *Yojo no Chie to Ki no Shiso* [Health Care and the Concept of Ki]. Kodansha Ltd.

栄西 Eisai. (1211- 1214). 喫茶養生記 *Kissa Yojoki* [Notes on Drinking Green Tea for Self-Care].

多田政一 Tada Masakazu. (1935). 綜統医学提唱論 *Soto Igaku Teishoron* [Integrated Medicine Advocacy]. Nihon Soto Gakujutsuin.

多田政一 Tada Masakazu. (1936). 綜統医学通説 *Soto Igaku Tsusetsu* [General Theory of Integrated Medicine]. Nihon Soto Gakujutsuin.

多田政一 Tada Masakazu. (1937). 科学より学問へ, *Kagaku yori Gakumon e*. Nihon Soto Gakujutsuin.

千島喜久男 Chishima Kikuo. (1985). 血液と健康の知恵―新血液理論と健康、治病への応用 医学革命の書 *Ketsueki to Kenko no Chie: Shin Ketsueki Riron to Kenko, Chibyo eno Oyo Igaku Kakumei no Sho* [Wisdom of Blood and Health: A Book of New Theory of Blood and Application to Health, Disease and Medical Revolution]. Jiyusha.

森下敬一 Morishita Keiichi. (1985). 自然医食で慢性病を克服する *Shizen Ishoku de Manseibyo wo Kokufuku suru*. [Overcoming Chronic Diseases with Natural Medicine Diet] Midori Shobo. Co., Ltd.

Further Readings

(1) Acupuncture

石原克己 Ishihara Katsumi. (2012, June 20). 意識と鍼灸 *Ishiki to Shinkyu*. 週刊あはき ワールド Shukan Ahaki World. Human world. <http://www.human-world.co.jp/ahaki_world/newsitem/12/0620/120620_1_ishiki.html>.

石原克己記 Ishihara Katsumi. 月刊東洋医学　東洋医学に何ができるか *Gekkan Toyo Igaku Toyo Igaku ni Nani ga Dekiruka*, Midori Shobo Co.,Ltd.

石原克己記 Ishihara Katsumi. 現代版素問 *Gendaiban Somon*. Gensosha.

石原克己 Ishihara Katsumi. 鍼灸と意識 *Shinkyu to Ishiki*. サトルエネルギー学会誌 第14 巻 通巻第26号 The Subtle Energy Association of Japan 14(26), 102-111.

石原克己 Ishihara Katsumi. 日々の臨床に役立つコツ *Hibi no Rinsho ni Yakudatsu Kotsu*. in 医道の日本社編集部 Ido no Nippon Sha Editorial staff. (eds.), 鍼灸臨床のコツ 002 Shinkyu Rinsho no Kotsu vol.2. (50-51). Ido no Nippon Sha.

浦山久嗣 Urayama Kyuzo. (2003). 六部定位脈診について *Rokubu Teii Myakushin ni tsuite*. 経絡治療 153, 154号 Keiro Chiryo 153, 154. Traditional Japanese Medicine.

源草社編 Gensosha. TAO鍼灸療法 *Tao Shinkyu Ryouhou*. Gensosha.

黄帝内経霊枢―現代語訳（上巻） *Huangdi Neijing Reisu Gendaigoyaku vol.1*. (1999). 南京中医学院中医系 Nankin Chui Gakuin Chuikei. (eds.), 石田秀実 Ishida Hidemi, 白杉悦雄 Shirasugi Etsuo (trans.), Toyo Gakujutsu Shuppansha.

黄帝内経霊枢―現代語訳（下巻） *Huangdi Neijing Reisu vol.2. Gendaigoyaku*. (2000). 南京中医学院中医系 Nankin Chui Gakuin Chuikei. (eds.), 石田秀実 Ishida Hidemi, 白杉悦雄 Shirasugi Etsuo and 前田繁樹 Maeda Shigeki. (trans.), Toyo Gakujutsu Shuppansha.

黄帝内経素問 上巻―現代語訳 *Huangdi Neijing Somon vol.1. Gendaigoyaku*. (1991). 南京中医学院中医系 Nankin Chui Gakuin Chuikei. (eds.), 島田隆司 Shimada Ryuji. (trans.), Toyo Gakujutsu Shuppansha.

黄帝内経素問 中巻―現代語訳 *Huangdi Neijing Somon vol.2. Gendaigoyaku*. (1992). 南京中医学院中医系 Nankin Chui Gakuin Chuikei. (eds.), 石田秀実 Ishida Hidemi. (trans.), Toyo Gakujutsu Shuppansha.

黄帝内経素問 下巻―現代語訳 *Huangdi Neijing Somon vol.3 Gendaigoyaku*. (1999). 南京中医学院中医系 Nankin Chui Gakuin Chuikei. (eds.), 石田秀実 Ishida Hidemi. (trans.), Toyo Gakujutsu Shuppansha.

長沢元夫 Nagasawa Motoo. 伝統医学の学び方 *Dento Igaku no Manabikata*. Sekibundo Shuppan.

長沢元夫 Nagasawa Motoo. 漢方鍼灸入門 *Kampo Shinkyu Nyumon*. Kyoeishobo.

長沢元夫博士の講演資料 *Nagasawa Motoo Hakese no Koen Shiryo*. 日本伝統医学協会 Nippon Dento Igaku Kyokai.

日中共同編集 Nicchu Kyodo Henshu. 針灸学(基礎篇) *Shinkyu Gaku(Kisohen)*. 東洋学術出版 Toyo Gakujutsu Shuppan.

臓腑学説の理論と運用 *Fuzo Gakusetsu no Riron to Unnyou*, 創医会学術部訳 Soikai Gakujutsubu

舟木寛伴 Funaki Hirotomo. 脈診へのいざない―身近なり、しかして深遠なり、脈診 *Myakushin eno Izanai Mijika nari, shikasite Shinen nari, Myakushin*. Taniguchi Shoten.

村山維益 Murayama Koremasu. 古脈法図解 *Komyakuhou Zukai*.

柳谷素霊 Yanagiya Sorei. 簡明不問診察法 *Kanmei Fumon Shinsatsuho*. Ishiyama Shinkyu Igakusha.

山下詢 Yamashita Makoto. 脈診入門六部定位脈診法 *Myakusin Nyumon Rokubu Teii Myakushinho*, Ishiyaku Shuppan.

山下詢 Yamashita Makoto. 鍼灸治療学 *Shinkyu Chiryou Gaku*. Ishiyaku Shuppan.

(2) Kampo

何任 Ka, Nin. 金匱要略解説 *Kingi Youryaku Kaisetsu*. Toyo Gakujyutsu Shuppansha.

長沢元夫 Nagasawa Motoo. 漢方薬物学入門 *kampo Yakubutsu Nyumon*. Chojyoshoten.

長沢元夫 Nagasawa Motoo. 現代人の漢方 *Gendaijin no kampo*. Toyokeizai Shinposha.

長沢元夫 Nagasawa Motoo. 新中国の漢方 *Shin Chugoku no kampo*. Shuppan Kagaku Sogo Kenkyujo.

日本漢方医学会 Nihon Kampo Igakukai. 漢方と漢薬 *Kampo to Kanyaku*. Shunyodo Shoten.

原南陽 Hara Nanyo. 近世漢方医学書集成19 *Kinsei kampo Igakusho Shuusei 19*. Meicho Shuppan.

平野重誠 Hirano Jusei. 病家須知 *Byo Ka Su Chi*. Rural Culture Association.

兪雪如他 Yu, Setsujyo. and et.al. 気血水 *Ki Ketsu Sui*. Taniguchi Shoten.

李時珍 Li, Jichin. 國譯本草綱目 Kokuyaku Honzo Komoku. Shunyodo Shoten.

(3) Dietary Care

石塚左玄 Ishizuka Sagen. 食物養生法 *Shokumotsu Yojo Ho*. Hakubunkan.

石塚左玄 Ishizuka Sagen. 食べ物健康法 *Tabemono Kenko Ho*. Rural Culture Association.

岡田周三 Okada Shuzo. 正食健康法入門 *Seishoku Kenko Nyumon*. Shinsensha.

久司道夫 Kushi Michio. マクロビオティック健康法 *Macrobiotic Kenko Ho*. Nichibou.

甲田光雄 Koda Mitsuo. 白砂糖の害は恐ろしい *Shirozato no Gai wa Osoroshii*. Ningen-igakusha.

桜沢如一 Sakurazawa Yukikazu. 東洋医学の哲学 *Toyo Igaku no Tetsugaku*. Japan CI Association.

桜沢如一 Sakurazawa Yukikazu. 無双原理・易 *Musou Genri,Eki*. Japan CI Association.

七田真 Shichida Makoto. あなたの子供はこんな危機にさらされている *Anata no Kodomo wa Konna Kiki ni Sarasareteiru*. Sogo Horei Publishing Co., Ltd.

外山利道 Toyama Toshimichi. 牛乳神話完全崩壊 *Gyunyu Shinwa Kanzen Houkai*. Metamoru Shuppan.

西勝造 Nishi Katsuzo. 西式健康法入門 *Nishi shiki Kenko Ho Nyumon*. Nishi kai Headquarters.

沼田勇 Numata Isamu. 病は食から *Yamai wa Shoku kara*. Rural Culture Association.

真弓定夫 Mayumi Sadao. アトピーっ子は治せる防げる *Atopic Ko wa Naoseru Fusegeru*. Ienohikari Association.

真弓定夫 Mayumi Sadao. 子供は病気を食べている *Kodomo wa Byouki wo Tabeteiru*. Ienohikari Association.

真弓定夫 Mayumi Sadao. 自然流育児のすすめ *Shizen Ryu Ikuji no Susume*. Jiyusha.

Walker, N. W. 生野菜汁療法 *Namayasai Jiru Ryoho*. Jitsugyo no Nihonsha.

(4) Psychology and Spiritual Healing

青木文紀 Aoki Fumirori. ヒーリング・ザ・レイキ―実践できる癒しのテクニック *Healing the Reiki: Jissen dekiru Iyashi no Technique*. Gensyuu Publishing. Co., Ltd.

伊豆山格堂 Izuyama Kakudo. 白隠禅師延命十句観音経霊験記 *Hakuin Zenji Enmei Jikku Kannon Gyo Reigenki*. Shunjusha.

井村宏次 Imura Koji. 霊術家の饗宴 *Reijutsuka no Kyoen*. Shinyusha.

上野正春 Ueno Masaharu. 神伝レイキの秘密: 今蘇る、幻の心身健康法「レイキ」: 日本が世界に誇るハンドヒーリングの最高峰「癒し～霊格向上～悟り」まで *Shinden Reiki no Himitsu: Ima Yomigaeru, Maboroshi no Shinshin Kenkoho 'Reiki' Nihon ga Sekai ni Hokoru Hand Healing no Saikoho 'Iyashi Reikakukojo Satori' Made*. Tama Publishing. Co., Ltd.

江口俊博 Eguchi Toshihiro. 三井甲之 Mitsui Koshi. 手のひら療法入門, *Tenohira Ryouhou Nyumon*. ARS.

大宮司朗 Omiya Shiro. 神通秘占神呪言霊玄修秘伝 *Jintsu Hisen Shinju Kotodama Genshu Hiden*. Hachiman Shoten.

大宮司朗 Omiya Shiro. 神法道術秘伝 *Shimpo Dojutsu Hiden*. Hachiman Shoten.

大宮司朗 Omiya Shiro. 神法妙術霊符 太古真法玄義 *Shimpo Myojutsu Reifu Taiko Simpo Gengi*, Hachiman Shoten.

大宮司朗 Omiya Shiro. 玄想法秘儀 *Gensoho Higi*. Hachiman Shoten.

大矢浩史 Oya Hiroshi. Oneness on the earth…地上の楽園〈vol.2〉こころの扉を開く旅 *Oneness on the earth…Chijo no Rakuen Vol.2: Kokoro no Tobira wo Hiraku Tabi*. Kalki Center Japan.

大山霊泉 Oyama Reisen. 霊掌術教授全書 *Reishojutsu Kyoju Zensho*. Hachiman Shoten.

岡野守也 Okano Moriya. トランスパーソナル心理学 *Transpersonal Shinri Gaku*. Seidosha.

柄澤照覚 Karasawa Shokaku. 神理療養強健術 *Shinri Ryoyo Kyokenjutsu*. Hachiman Shoten.

川面凡兒 Kawatsura Bonji. 大日本最古の神道：川面凡児選集 *Dainihon Saiko no Shinto: Kawatsuwa Bonji Senshu*. Hachiman Shoten.

河野良和 Kono Yoshikazu. 催眠療法入門 *Saimin Ryoho Nyumon*. Kono Shinri Kenkyujo.

小林信子 Kobayashi Nobuko. 岡田虎二郎先生語録 *Okada Torajiro Sensei Goroku*. Seizasha.

渋川玄耳 Shibukawa Genji. 神仙 *Shinsen*. Hachiman Shoten.

滝澤朋子 Takizawa Tomoko. あなたも魔法使いになれるホ・オポノポノ *Anata mo Mahoutsukai ni Nareru Ho'oponopono*. Total health design.

岸根卓郎 Takuro Kishine. 宇宙の意思―人は何処より来りて、何処へ去るか *Uchu no Ishi_ Hito wa Doko yori Kitarite, Doko e Saruka*. Toyo Keizai Shimposha.

田中守平 Tanaka Morihei. 太霊道及霊子術講義録(上下巻) *Taireido oyobi Reishijutsu Kogiroku Vol.1 and 2*. Hachiman Shoten.

常岡一郎 Tsuneoka Ichiro. 中心百巻, *Chushin Hyakkan*. Chushinsha.

常岡一郎 Tsuneoka Ichiro. 天の手紙(上・中・下), *Ten no Tegami Vol.1, 2 and 3*. Chushinsha.

天外伺朗, Tenge Shiiro. 理想的な死に方―「あの世」の科学が死・生・魂の概念を変えた! *Risoteki na Shinikata_'Anoyo' no Kagaku Ga Shi Sei Tamashii no Gainen wo Kaeta!*. 徳間書店 Tokuma Shoten.

土居裕 Doi Hiroshi. 癒しの現代霊気法：伝統技法と西洋式レイキの神髄 *Iyashi no Gendai Reikiho: Dentogiho to Seiyoushiki Reiki no Shinzui*. Gensyuu Publishing. Co., Ltd.

徳山暉純 Tokuyama Kijyun. 梵字手帳 *Bonji Techo*. Mokujisha.

富田魁二 Tomida Kaiji. 霊気と仁術~富田流手あて療法 *Reiki to Jinjutsu Tomidaryu Teateryoho*. BAB JAPAN Co., Ltd.

直木公彦 Naoki Kimihiko. 白隠禅師―健康法と逸話 *Hakuin Zenji Kenkohou to Itsuwa*. Nippon Kyoubunsha.

西勝造 Nishi Katsuzo. 原本・西式健康読本, *Gempon Nishi Shiki Kenko Dokuhon*. Rural Culture Association Japan.

西村大観 Nishimura Taikan. 西村式霊術叢書 *Nishimura Shiki Reijutsu Sosho*. Hachimanshoten.

平田内蔵吉 Hirata Kurakichi. 触手中心健康法 *Shokushu Chushin Kenkoho*. Sangakusha.

Becker, Carl. B., 柏木哲夫 Kashiwagi Tetsuo and *et.al.* 潔く死ぬために *Isagiyoku Shinutameni*. Shunjusha Publishing Company.

松原皎月 Matsubara Kogetsu. 自然運動法; 催眠術講義 *Shizen Undoho; Saiminjutsu Kogi*. Hachiman Shoten.

松原皎月 Matsubara Kogetsu. 神傳靈學奥義 *Shinden Reigaku Ogi*. Senshinkai.

松原皎月 Matsubara Kogetsu. 霊熱透射療法秘傳書; 診断法虎之巻 *Reinetsutosha Ryoho Hidensho: Shindanho Toranomaki*. Senshinkai.

松本道別 Matsumoto Dobetsu. 霊学講座, *Reigaku Koza*. Hachiman Shoten.

三浦一郎 Miura Ichiro. 奇蹟のハンド・ヒーリング―あなたの手に隠された超エネルギーの活用, *Kiseki no Hand Healing_ Anata no Te ni Kakusareta Cho Energy no Katsuyo*. Tama Publishing. Co., Ltd.

武藤安孝 Muto Yasutaka. 安全マスター催眠術 *Anzen Master Saimin Jutsu*. Bungei Shuppan.

村上和雄 Murakami Kazuo. 遺伝子からのメッセージ *Idenshi Kara no Message*. Asahibunko.

村上和雄 Murakami Kazuo. 人生の暗号 *Jinsei no Ango*. Sunmark Publishing. Inc.

村上和雄 Murakami Kazuo. 生命の暗号 *Inochi no Ango*. Sunmark Publishing. Inc.

吉田弘 Yoshida Hiroshi. 手の妙用：大自然の治癒力 *Te no Myoyo*: Daishizen no Chiyuryoku. Tomeisha.

Cummins, Geraldine. *The Road to Immortality*. White Crow Books.

Frager, Robert and Fadiman, James. *Personality and Personal Growth*. Joanna Cotler Books.

Hay, House. *You Can Heal Your Life*. Hay House Inc.

Krasner, A. M. *The Wizard within: The Krasner Method of Hypnotherapy*. American Board of Hydrotherapy Press

Krishnamurti, J. *The First and Last Freedom*. Rider & Co.

Kubis, Pat. and Macy, Mark. *Conversations Beyond the Light: Communication with Departed Friends & Colleagues by Electronic Means*. Griffin Pub Group.

Kübler-Ross, Elisabeth. *On Death and Dying*. Routledge.

Muller, Brigitte. and Gunther, Horst. H. *A Complete Book of Reiki Healing*. Basic Health Publications, Inc.

Myss, Caroline. *Anatomy of the Spirit: The Seven Stages of Power and Healing*. Harmony.

Myss, Caroline. *Why People Don't Heal and How They Can*. *H*armony.

Page, Christine, R. *Frontiers of Health: How to Heal the Whole Person*. Random House.

Pearson, E. Norman. *Space, Time and Self (illustrated)*. Theosophical Pub. House.

Roberts, Jane. and Butts, R. Freeman. *Seth Speaks: The Eternal Validity of the Soul. Amber-Allen Publ., New World Library.*

Rose, Linda. Joy. *Your Mind: The Owner's Manual.* Kriya Yoga Publications.

Sarno, John. E. *Healing Back Pain,* Grand Central Publishing.

Steiner, Rudolf. *Die Offenbarungen des Karma,* Rudolf Steiner Verlag.

(6)Others

新村出 Shimmura Izuru. 広辞苑 第四版 普通版 *Kojien Daiyonban Futsu ban.* Iwanami Shoten. Publishers.

千島喜久男 Chishima Kikuo. 血液と健康の知恵―新血液理論と健康、治病への応用 医学革命の書 *Ketsueki to Kenko no Chie_Shin ketsueki Riron to Kenko, Chibyo eno Oyo Igaku Kakumei no Sho.* Jiyusha.

千島喜久男 Chishima Kikuo. 女性文明待望論 *Josei Bummei Taiboron.* Shin Seimei Igaku kai.

千島喜久男 Chishima Kikuo. 千島学説論争 *Chishima Gakusetsu Ronso.* Shin Seimei Igaku kai.

千島喜久男 Chishima Kikuo. 文明と生命＿物質文明と生命の没落 *Bummei to Seimei _ Busshitsu Bummei to Seimei no Botsuraku.* Shin Ketsueki Gakkai.

西原克成 Nishihara Katsunari. 「赤ちゃん」の進化学: 子供を病気にしない育児の科学 *'Akachan' no Shinkagaku: Kodomo wo Byoki ni Shinai Ikuji no Kagaku.* Kobunsha Co., Ltd.

日本母乳の会 Nipppon Bonyu no Kai. 卒乳―おっぱいはいつまで*Sotsunyu Oppai wa itsumade.* Nipppon Bonyu no Kai.

Capra, Fritjof. *The Turning Point: Science, Society, and the Rising Culture.* Fontana.

Carrel, Alexis. *Man, the Unknown.* Burns & Oates Ltd.

Chopra, Deepak. *Quantum Healing: Exploring the Frontiers of Mind/Body Medicine.* Bantam.

Luke, Matthew. *New Testament.*

Madaus, Gerhard. *Lehrbuch der biologischen Heilmittel.* Thieme.

Samuel, Foreword. *Job Book: Old Testament.*